THE
Setpoint
DIET

THE
Setpoint
DIET

The 21-Day Program to Permanently Change
What Your Body "Wants" to Weigh

JONATHAN BAILOR

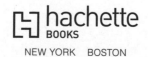

hachette
BOOKS

NEW YORK   BOSTON

Hachette Books
Hachette Book Group
1290 Avenue of the Americas
New York, NY 10104
hachettebooks.com
twitter.com/hachettebooks

First Edition: December 2018

Hachette Books is a division of Hachette Book Group, Inc.
The Hachette Books name and logo are trademarks of Hachette Book Group, Inc.

The publisher is not responsible for websites (or their content) that are not owned by the publisher.

The Hachette Speakers Bureau provides a wide range of authors for speaking events. To find out more, go to www.hachettespeakersbureau.com or call (866) 376-6591.

Library of Congress Cataloging-in-Publication Data

Names: Bailor, Jonathan, author.
Title: The setpoint diet : the 21-day program to permanently change
    what your body "wants" to weigh / Jonathan Bailor.
Description: First edition. | New York, NY : Hachette Books, 2019. | Includes
    bibliographical references and index.
Identifiers: LCCN 2018026343| ISBN 9780316483834 (hardcover) | ISBN 9781549141263
    (audio download) | ISBN 9780316483841 (ebook)
Subjects: LCSH: Reducing diets. | Weight loss. | Metabolism. | Nutrition. | Exercise.
Classification: LCC RM222.2 .B3447 2019 | DDC 613.2/5—dc23
LC record available at https://lccn.loc.gov/2018026343

Printed in the United States of America

LSC-H

10 9 8 7 6 5 4 3 2 1

To my beloved Angela.
May our perfect partnership continue to manifest miracles.

To the SANE Family.
Thank you for being the change we want to see in the world. You are taking the road less traveled and it will make all the difference.

To my father, Robert, and mother, Mary Rose.
All that is good finds its origins in your love.

To my daughter, Aavia Gabrielle.
We will create a SANEr world for you. I promise.

CONTENTS

INTRODUCTION

Your Weight Is Not Your Fault

Inside that beautiful body of yours is a naturally thin person struggling to come out—someone who can eat as much as he or she wants, does not need to spend hours exercising, and can still stay slim. You know people like that. Maybe you've envied them. Maybe you've wished your body worked like theirs.

Until now, you've been forever fighting against your body and your mind. You've determined your worth by a number on the scale. You've held yourself to impossibly high standards that do nothing but fester inside you and make you feel hopeless.

Get ready for a different approach.

With the Setpoint Diet, there will be no more exhausting fights with yourself. I'm offering you a new approach that works *with* your body and mind to help you become naturally thin.

Can you imagine what that would be like? Just think: Never dieting. Never feeling like you must make up for nutritional sins. Instead, your body effortlessly burns calories all day long, rather than stores them as fat. You stop losing and regaining the same 20, 50, or more pounds over and over again throughout your life. You maintain a healthy, empowering weight—and even enjoy some cheesecake or French fries every now and then without worrying about putting on *any* pounds.

I'm here to tell you that you can be a member of that exclusive "club" of naturally thin people. In fact, I'm handing you your membership card right now. I realize that it sounds too good to be true. But it is the truth—and scores of scientific studies, plus tens of thousands of success stories prove it...and you will have proven it for yourself less than 30 days from now.

You see, there's an *invisible force* inside you that is conspiring to cling to extra pounds, and it has nothing to do with calories, points, mail-order meals, cardiovascular exercise, or any of the conventional diet nonsense you've been fed—and that has failed you over and over for most of your life.

What's truly holding you back—and what can permanently set you free—can be summed up in a word: *setpoint*. And it's something you can control. When you control it, you stay naturally thin.

WHAT IS A SETPOINT?

In a nutshell, *setpoint* refers to the level of stored fat the body works to maintain by regulating your appetite and metabolism through your hormones, genes, and brain, regardless of the quantity of calories you take in or exercise off.

Setpoint also explains why you have such a tough time keeping fat off through traditional diet and exercise programs. Think of it as a clogged sink. What if your plumber came in and said the cure for the clog was to stop using your sink? Sure, this fixes the symptom (the sink's not going to overflow) but not the cause (what's causing the clog?). And who wants dirty hands for the rest of their life?! The cause of that clog is eating poor-quality foods and establishing habits that throw your fat-burning, appetite-taming hormones out of whack.

This plan is about lowering your setpoint in order to keep your body in a fat-burning mode 24/7. When this happens, you also KEEP those pounds off. Every day of your life, you will wake up in the type of body that you deserve and that has previously seemed impossible to achieve.

I know this is a lot to take in. But understand that we all have a setpoint— and that's what determines how thin or overweight we are LONG-TERM. *Not calorie-counting or traditional forms of exercising.* When you increase the quality of your eating, exercise, and habits, you lower your setpoint—and get your body to burn fat rather than store it.

That's what *The Setpoint Diet* is all about. It removes the willpower, shame, and guilt from the weight and diabetes equation. It ends the frustration and the yo-yo dieting. It stops the painful and expensive health consequences of diabesity, and does it with a proven system that will set the naturally thin person inside you free once and for all.

You are going to learn science and strategies—and apply them to your life—that are going to be radically counter to what you've heard before but are guaranteed to be absolutely life-changing. You will have to try some things you've never done before. You will have to let go of old beliefs about eating and self-incrimination over failed dieting and make the decision to create the body and the health you desire like your life depends on it.

And honestly, your life does depend on it. And you are worth it. Really, you are.

MY SETPOINT STORY

One of my earliest and most painful memories is watching my grandfather endure heartbreaking and completely avoidable suffering. He was a superhero to me—a second-generation American with parents who spoke no English. He never graduated from high school, yet instilled in his four children the power of education. All four went on to get master's degrees or higher.

For all he achieved in his life—from earning respect in the community to raising a beautiful, brilliant family—his superpowers could not help him overcome a supervillain that threatens more than one out of every four of us: diabetes.

When my grandfather's leg became septic due to complications of diabetes, he was rushed to the hospital. Surgeons advised that his leg be amputated to save his life. But he would not agree to this surgery.

From outside his hospital room, I heard him calling to my mother, who was at his bedside. "Please don't let them take my leg...please don't!"

My family decided to honor my grandfather's wishes and steadfastly refused the lifesaving operation. He kept both legs, but within 48 hours, he was gone.

Diabetes took him from us just as diabetes is taking so many more of us and so many of our loved ones. To this day, every year, the dual epidemics of obesity and diabetes—"diabesity"—kill more people than smoking, alcohol, and drugs combined.

When people ask me why I got into the business of teaching others how to lose weight and get healthier *permanently*, I tell them the story of my grandfather—and how I pledged to make sure that the superheroes in our lives don't fall victim to lifestyle diseases the same way he did.

Growing up, I idolized two more superheroes. The first was the Man of Steel himself: Superman. In fact, my mother can tell you stories about my refusal to wear anything other than this outfit:

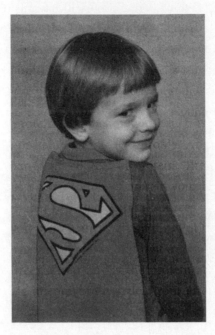

The second superhero was my big brother, a strong, muscular football player. Every night, I'd sit at the dinner table with him and my brainy college professor parents, dreaming of the day when I would be as strong as he was. But as birthdays came and went, the opposite happened—I grew lankier, not bigger and stronger.

So I did what any professors' kid would do: I studied, devouring every health and fitness magazine and book under the sun, and listening to big, strong men like my brother talk about how to get big and strong. I thought I had finally discovered the secret to becoming Superman. After I went to college, I decided to put some of this hard-earned knowledge to work and help other people change their bodies as a personal trainer.

Every day, I counted calories, all the way up to 6,000 daily because I wanted to bulk up. I asked my clients to count calories, too, but so they could lose weight. Those clients were some of the most amazing, health-savvy women and men I have ever met: CEOs, doctors, and teachers. At first, I advised them to eat 1,600 calories daily and exercise for half an hour each day. But they couldn't lose a pound, despite their successes in business and in life. So I cut their food intake down to 1,400 calories and increased their workouts to an hour a day. That didn't work either. I slashed their diets down to 1,200 calories a day and upped their exercising to 90 minutes daily. Their weight still didn't budge. As for me, I didn't gain a single ounce of muscle.

I wasn't gaining weight eating 6,000 calories per day, and my clients, even on such restricted diets, weren't losing weight—we were all just getting sick and depressed.

What was the problem? I assumed it was that we just needed to try harder. I guess I should eat 8,000 calories per day and my clients should eat 800.

One day, while I knocked back a shot of calorie-packed olive oil, it suddenly occurred to me: What if some big strong man out there was thinking the exact same thing about me? "If that skinny, geeky kid could just eat more, he would gain weight—what's his problem? He just needs to try harder."

In a flash, I realized that even though all I'd ever wanted to do was to help people feel healthier and better about themselves, what I was doing was making everyone—including myself—sicker and sadder. By urging them to try harder, I was making them feel more guilt and shame.

I stopped training clients because I realized that advising them to count calories and overexercise was hurting them.

After making so many mistakes, I was hell-bent on making things right, so I asked my college professor parents for advice. I told them about the countless hours I'd spent reading and studying and applying what I'd learned—and the results I wasn't seeing. They said, "You and your clients are not suffering from an effort problem. You're all trying really hard. What you have is an information problem. Consider the sources."

They were absolutely correct. So I discarded everything I thought I knew and started fresh, beginning a new journey that took me deep into the foreign lands of jargon-packed scientific studies and mind-bending academic journal articles. In the process, I discovered that everything I'd ever been taught as a trainer was disproven in the scientific literature. What I thought I knew about fitness and weight loss was wrong.

As I learned more, I was no longer interested in fighting against the body; I wanted to learn how to transform the body. I wanted to find out how to improve the system itself rather than use barbaric starvation or obsessive exercise to torture people with a system that wasn't working correctly in the first place. Fifteen years, 10,000 pages of research, 1,300 scientific studies, and countless conversations with scientists later, I emerged from my research journey reborn.

For the first time, I realized a powerful truth: I would never be "strong enough" to leap tall buildings in a single bound. My genes simply wouldn't allow it. But I also realized a truth that freed me and changed my life forever: While I might never become Superman, I could become, through modern nutrition and exercise science, the very best version of the person I was born to be.

And that is exactly what will happen to you: You'll become the healthiest, happiest, most energetic super-version of you.

Once I realized how the body really works—through the proven new science of slim—I couldn't wait to share the information with the world. I recommitted my life to helping people achieve their weight-loss and health goals with data and facts, rather than hurting them with fairy tales of starvation dieting and extreme exercise.

Since the beginning of my research journey more than 15 years ago, I went on to lead multiple development teams at Microsoft, registered 25 patents, and had wonderful opportunities to work with some of the most well-known products in the fitness industry, including the Nike+ Kinect Training platform and Xbox Fitness. I merged my learning in the realm of biology and exercise physiology with my engineering background, to literally engineer solutions for fitness and nutrition. And so with this book, I share tools with you that will save your life if you take action and put them into use. You can literally re-engineer your body into the body of a naturally thin person, and I'll show you how.

The bottom line is, you can transform your body. And it's easier than you think. You can eat more, not less—and you will get leaner and healthier in the process. You can enjoy an astounding level of energy, vibrancy, love, and satisfaction in your life—without spending most of it in a gym. You don't have to suffer. You just need the correct information and the right guidance. And good news: You will get all of that here.

I want to help you realize how wonderful you are, to understand the strength, courage, and capability that have been gifted to you but have yet to be taken out of the box. It's a choice, and you can make it. You can decide: This is my time to live the very best life possible. No longer will I wait. No longer will I sit on the bench watching other people fulfill their dreams. This is the time when I will live the life I was meant to live! This is my time to transform! This is when I will go SANE (Satiety, Aggression, Nutrition, and Efficiency).

That life is here for you right now. Thank you for the privilege and honor of sharing it with you.

SANEly,

Jonathan Bailor
Seattle, Washington

PART 1

THE HIDDEN KEY TO LASTING
WEIGHT LOSS: YOUR SETPOINT

CHAPTER 1

Unlock the Naturally Thin You

You've been on diet after diet.

You've cut calories, carbs, and fat.

You've exercised your heart out.

You've lost weight, maybe a lot of it. But you gained it back, over and over again. Nothing you do works. You can't seem to drop pounds, nor can you keep them off.

What gives?

It all goes back to setpoint—the weight your body will try to maintain no matter what sort of "diet" you try. The only way to lose weight and keep it off is to lower your setpoint.

The Setpoint Diet is an empowering plan (the opposite of an "elimination diet") for eating and living that will unlock the naturally thin person inside you, so that you can enjoy your ideal weight permanently. It will reshape your body and the way you think about weight loss—no more cutting calories or torturing yourself with exercise you hate; no more feeling tired, hungry, and defeated all the time.

Always remember that you are not to blame for any weight issue you may be experiencing. I know you might not truly accept this yet, but it's true. Right now, please pause for a second and repeat out loud: "I am not to blame for my weight."

Because of the wrong information and the resulting societal misunderstanding about overweight and obesity, you've been guilted, shamed, and bullied into trying to lose weight with terribly wrong, hurtful advice: Just do it, stop being lazy, get your act together. Sadly, a lot of this "body shaming" or "fat shaming" comes from people and groups who should know better—nutritionists, psychologists, stick-thin celebrities. This is so wrong and unfair. For one thing, estimates of heritability of obesity and overweight range from 30 to 70 percent, with the typical

3

estimate at 50 percent, according to a report published in the *Journal of Clinical Nutrition* (Lyon and Hirschhorn 2005). So are many diseases such as diabetes, heart disease, and cancer. All of these, including obesity, should be treated with respect and consideration. Sadly, those "experts" didn't get that memo.

Fat shaming and bullying will never help you or anyone else lose weight. It only urges you to feel ashamed, rather than empowered. A study in the *American Journal of Public Health* underscores the suffering and shame that overweight people in our society face. It pointed out that 8 out of 10 people who are overweight or obese avoid going out in public for fear of being bullied over their appearance (Puhl and Heurer 2010). People who suffer from the chronic diseases overweight, obesity, and diabetes deserve the same compassion and scientific solutions provided to people suffering from more "socially acceptable" chronic diseases such as cancer or heart disease.

This brutality is further compounded when you're told to do things that just don't work, such as eating less, exercising more, and trying harder—all of which have a documented failure rate of 95.4 percent (Crawford 2000). Plus, these unworkable actions create another loop of guilt, shame, low self-esteem, depression, and more difficulty in keeping weight under control.

The beautiful thing is that hurt, suffering, shame, and other negative emotions do not exist in this book or in any of its supporting tools. Instead, you are going to patiently, permanently, and persistently heal your body, mind, and spirit—using a proven plan that solves weight as a scientific problem, rather than a character fault.

Whether you need to lose a few extra pounds around your waistline or you are looking for a complete body transformation, you are finally in the right place. The starting point of this journey is looking more closely at "setpoint weight"— the greatest determining factor in how much you weigh.

WHAT IS SETPOINT WEIGHT?

The human body is a beautifully complex biological machine. Your brain, your digestive system, and your hormones all work together through a highly coordinated system to help stabilize your weight—the same way they automatically stabilize your body temperature, blood pressure, and blood sugar.

Your brain, digestive system, and hormones talk to one another through various feedback loops to synchronize the activities that automatically maintain body fat at a specific level, otherwise known as your setpoint weight.

Think of the biological feedback system that establishes your setpoint weight like the thermostat in your house. Thanks to the thermostat, your heating or air-conditioning system responds to the weather outside and keeps your home at whatever temperature the thermostat "thinks" it should be at. Similarly, your setpoint stimulates or suppresses your appetite and raises or lowers metabolism—your body's food-to-fuel process—in response to how much fat it "thinks" you should store.

Let's say you decide to lose weight—and you go on some sort of starvation diet. After all, that's what you've been taught to do all these years, right? The story goes that if you reduce 500 calories a day, you're going to lose 3,500 calories by the end of the week—which is the equivalent of 1 pound. Do this for a couple of months and—bang—you've dropped about 8 pounds.

Sadly, your personal dieting experience (and decades of it!) coupled with modern science proves it doesn't work this way—*at all*—and this is because of your setpoint. When you start to cut calories, your body's metabolic alarm goes off (just like a thermostat responds when outside temperatures nose-dive to freezing). It signals your body—which strives for *homeostasis* or that stable status quo—that you are not consuming as much as you normally do. In response, your body demands more food and starts burning fewer calories. Appetite goes up, calorie burn goes down. This is why it seems like your body fights you every step of the way when you try to lose weight—because it does.

So you see, your weight is all about your setpoint! With each "cycle" of this plan, you'll lower your setpoint weight 10 pounds until you reach your ideal healthy setpoint. No matter how elevated your setpoint has become, this plan will engineer your body to burn fat like a naturally thin person so that you can effortlessly enjoy a body that looks and feels its best.

Once you see the science of setpoint weight, you can see how offensive it is to tell people who struggle with obesity that they "aren't trying hard enough." Telling people who suffer from an elevated setpoint to eat less and exercise more is like telling depressed people to frown less and smile more. Science has proven that both "light" and "heavy" bodies are abiding by the same science of the setpoint—"heavy" individuals just happen to have an elevated setpoint.

In fact, research over the last 30 years has shown exactly what I am describing: If you have an elevated setpoint, your body will fight to hold on to extra fat for its own survival. Let's take a look at some of this science right now.

THE SETPOINT SCIENCE OF "CALORIE MATH"

Fifteen years ago, when I embarked on this journey to uncover the truth about how dieting makes us heavy, sick, and sad, I didn't know just how many hours I would spend poring over study after study (I ended up at around 1,300—and counting—which you can see at SANESolution.com/Bibliography). Nor did I realize how much resistance I would encounter from non-medical "experts" and companies trying to hold us hostage with blatant lies and confusing messages about how complicated it must be to live a healthy and happy life.

Once you understand how your setpoint works (and how to hit *your* ideal setpoint), you'll see that all that other weight-loss methods are just nonsense.

What I will share with you in this section is the nuts and bolts of setpoint science. There's no need for you to spend 15 years plowing through all the studies like I did; I'm giving you the summary highlights. This information will begin to set you free. Ready?

Scientists who are studying the concept of setpoint start by asking themselves two questions:

1. If you eat more calories, does your body automatically burn more calories?
2. If you eat fewer calories, does your body automatically burn fewer calories?

Every study that has ever asked either of these questions has shown that both of these statements are true. Further, every relevant study ever conducted has shown that if fed too many (or too few) calories, people don't gain as much weight as "calorie math" would predict. Why? Their setpoint "fought back" to try to keep the study participants at what it "thought" they should weigh.

One of the earliest studies to demonstrate the concept of a setpoint weight was done in 1995 by a team of scientists at New York's Rockefeller University. They proved that metabolism disproportionately slows down after pounds have been shed—and that the metabolism remains slow, even after the "diet" is over. The researchers, led by Rudolph L. Leibel, studied 18 overweight volunteers and 23 people who had never been obese. The results, published in 1995 in the *New England Journal of Medicine*, showed that the obese and the lean respond to weight changes the same way. When they lost 10 percent of their body weight, their bodies compensated by burning up 15 percent fewer calories than would be expected. When they increased their weight by 10 percent, they used up 15 percent more calories (Leibel et al. 1995).

Based on these findings, Leibel and his colleagues believed they had identified an internal control (now known as setpoint) that tries to keep body fat at a reasonably constant level. This level differs from person to person, but how the body works to maintain it—adjusting metabolism in response to both weight loss and gain—is the same in everyone. If you start taking pounds off by eating less, your metabolism slows. If you start putting pounds on by eating more, your metabolism speeds up.

Here's another example: As reported in *Science*, researchers at the Mayo Clinic fed people 1,000 extra calories per day for 8 weeks. A thousand extra calories per day for 8 weeks totals 56,000 extra calories. But nobody gained 16 pounds—56,000 calories' worth—of body fat. The most anyone gained was a little over half that. And some participants gained basically nothing—less than a pound (Levine et al. 1999).

How can 56,000 extra calories add up to nothing?

It's because extra calories don't *have* to turn into body fat. They can be burned off automatically. This has been known in the scientific community for nearly a century. For example, in 1932 the *Quarterly Journal of Medicine* reported, "Food in excess of immediate requirements...can easily be disposed of, being burnt up and dissipated as heat. Did this capacity not exist, obesity would be almost universal" (Lyon and Dunlop 1932).

Eating more and gaining less is possible because when you have a lower setpoint, your body has all sorts of little-known ways to deal with surplus calories other than storing them as body fat. In the Mayo Clinic study, researchers measured three of them:

1. Your body can increase the amount of calories it burns daily (your "base metabolic rate").
2. Your body can increase the amount of calories it burns digesting food.
3. Your body can increase the amount of calories it burns via unconscious activity—little movements like shifting in your chair or fidgeting with your pen that some of us are more prone to than others.

Here is what they found:

Daily Response to 1,000 Extra Calories

	High Setpoint	Low Setpoint
Base Calories Burned Daily	Decreased by 100 calories	Increased by 360 calories
Calories Burned Digesting Food	Increased by 28 calories	Increased by 256 calories
Calories Burned via Unconscious Activity	Decreased by 98 calories	Increased by 692 calories
Total Daily Response	**Burned 170 Fewer Calories**	**Burned 1,308 More Calories**

That is how some people ate 56,000 extra calories without gaining any weight. A lower setpoint does its best to automatically balance more calories in with more calories out by upping the calories you burn as your base metabolic rate, when digesting food, and through unconscious activity.

A few years ago, the role of setpoint and metabolism took center stage after the release of shocking research involving 16 contestants on NBC's hit show *The Biggest Loser*, in which people diagnosed with obesity are publicly tortured into losing the most weight possible as quickly as possible (Fothergill et al. 2016).

Researchers discovered that 6 years after competing in the show, contestants' bodies had adapted to their weight loss with a disproportionately *decreased* metabolic rate that persisted for years. Essentially, their bodies were working all day, every day, to regain the lost weight by driving their appetite and cravings up and their metabolisms down. When participants cut calories to maintain their new, thinner physiques, their metabolism slowed down even more. Eventually, their bodies were burning so few calories that most people were doomed to gain back all the weight they lost, and then some.

In these, and every case of "eat less, exercise more," the contestants' setpoint kicked in. No matter how drastically they cut calories, their setpoint overrode their weight-loss efforts and returned them to higher weights and greater preservation of fat stores.

I worked with two former *Biggest Loser* contestants, Jay and Jennifer. While on this show, Jennifer temporarily lost 114 pounds, and Jay temporarily lost 181 pounds. Weight lost via dietary and physical torture is not effective or entertaining—it's metabolically damning—so it is no wonder that once the show ended, the pounds started coming back.

Jay and Jennifer told me, "Our bodies seem to have minds of their own."

Indeed, that "mind" was their setpoint. Jay and Jennifer had temporarily lost weight by forcing their body to stray from its setpoint, but since they had not lowered the setpoint itself, the second they stopped fighting against their bodies, all the weight came right back. As Jay told me: "I've lost 100 pounds a bunch of times. Temporary weight loss is not the issue. Keeping it off is the issue."

Jay and Jennifer then used the tools you will learn in *The Setpoint Diet*. After following the plan for just 30 days, they were thriving and told me that they felt they had achieved their "personal best." That's because they were working with their bodies instead of fighting a losing battle against their setpoints.

THE PROBLEM OF AN ELEVATED SETPOINT

An elevated setpoint makes KEEPING weight off practically impossible, but why?

Every cell in your body is designed to keep you alive and requires proper nutrition to do that. So when you give your cells less nutrition than they "think" they need, they interpret that as nothing short of slow death. If you attempt to starve your way to weight-loss success, you must fight every cell in your body every second of every day.

And the disappointing reality is that the more often and severely you starve yourself, the harder your body will fight to protect any and all fat in the future. Starvation dieting literally turns your body into a fat-storing, fat-protecting machine. Even when you are no longer technically starving, your body will overreact to prevent that "famine" from ever happening again by increasing your setpoint. As long as your setpoint stays elevated, one of three things must happen:

1. You starve pounds away, then stop starving yourself, and all the pounds return and stay put even more stubbornly than before.

2. You starve the pounds away, and then spend every waking hour of your life waging an unwinnable war against yourself by eating fewer and fewer calories with each passing year to maintain the weight loss.

3. You resign yourself to "never" having the body, energy, or health you desire.

Sound like something you can relate to?

But what if you got the power of your setpoint working *for* you rather than *against* you? Then, just like every cell in your body once worked to store calories as fat, *now* they work to burn calories. And spoiler alert: That's exactly what the Setpoint Diet will do for you! Lower your setpoint and you lower your weight *permanently.*

Now equipped with your lower setpoint, go back to that seemingly hopeless list, and check out the transformed future waiting for you:

1. You eat more, your body burns more, and your weight stays at your lower setpoint.
2. You eat the same amount and your weight stays at your lower setpoint.
3. You eat less (I'm not sure why you'd do this, but let's be comprehensive here), your body burns less, and your weight returns to your lower setpoint.

In short, no matter what you do, your body works to keep you at an ideal weight as diligently as it had worked to keep you overweight. Plus, you now have proof that your weight says nothing about a lack of effort or willpower or even character flaws, because you've been given gimmicky tools and fad diets for weight loss and have *increased* your setpoint weight. You fight a losing battle against your setpoint and can't possibly give you anything more than *short-term* weight loss followed by long-term weight gain. Game changer, no?

Here is a closer look.

Your Body Defends Its Fat Stores

As we touched on before, one reason the body maintains a higher setpoint is because you need a certain amount of fat to live. Fat plays a role in every single cell in your body, plus a big role in the functioning of your nervous system and in the absorption of many nutrients. Besides the global role of fat in your body, fat tissue itself functions as an endocrine (hormone-secreting) organ. It preserves a setpoint-determined level of fat on your body that your brain "thinks" is best for you.

This means that on the last starvation diet you tried, your brain went into crisis mode for lack of nutrition (vitamins, minerals, etc.) and energy (calories).

Through many different hormonal feedback mechanisms, your brain knows if you are not taking in enough nutrition to maintain what it "thinks" you should weigh, and it will instruct your body to burn as few calories as possible and store as many calories as possible as body fat.

That's only part of the story. To make sure that your setpoint stays stable, the body starts looking around for other sources of energy. And it invariably turns to muscle. This is your most metabolically active tissue, which means it uses up a lot of energy just to maintain on a daily basis. If you are not feeding your body sufficient amounts of energy, it is going to start breaking down muscle to feed the fat stores. When muscle starts burning off, your body gets listless, less healthy, and surprisingly, *fatter* on the inside. With less muscle, your setpoint creeps up even higher.

When you starve yourself, your body prefers to break down more muscle for fuel. You are literally eating yourself alive. You can try to cut calories all you want, but until you address the underlying cause—an elevated setpoint—your body will find the calories it needs, especially by burning off calorie-hungry muscle.

Not only does setpoint explain why it's so hard to keep fat off by eating less and exercising more, but it also explains why people do not keep getting heavier and heavier until they explode. I know this sounds silly, but seriously, why doesn't someone who weighs 450 pounds eventually eat their way up to 4,500 pounds?

Again, the answer lies in the setpoint. Most obese people hold a stable weight around their elevated setpoint. As researcher D. S. Weigle at the University of Washington points out: "[O]besity is not a disorder of body weight regulation. Most obese patients regulate their weight appropriately about an elevated setpoint weight" (Weigle 1990).

Obesity is simply the result of the body being good at defending its fat and its elevated weight. A heavy person's higher setpoint prompts the body to store more fat for the same reason that a thin person's lower setpoint prompts the body to burn more fat. That's why I couldn't gain weight eating 6,000 calories while my clients couldn't lose weight eating 1,200 calories.

Yo-Yo Dieting Can Elevate Setpoint

The counterproductive nature of starvation dieting—like the methods Jay and Jennifer initially tried—is what scientists call "weight cycling," or more simply "yo-yo dieting." This refers to losing weight, then gaining more back.

If you are like 95.4 percent of dieters, there's a good chance that you have experience with this cycle. You go on a diet, you shed pounds, then you stop starving yourself, and you gain it all back and more. Losing the weight was easy; keeping it off was hard, so the weight—and then some—comes back on.

Studies prove that regaining weight after starvation dieting is no more your fault than shivering when you're cold is your fault. Both are how the human body protects itself from harm. You may want to write this down, as it can save your life: Starvation isn't healthy; it's deadly.

Now, sadly, unlike how it protects itself from freezing to death (goose bumps, shivering, and so forth), your body's defense against starving to death—yo-yo dieting and setpoint elevation—has a long-term impact. The explanation goes something like this: Let's say you weigh 200 pounds. Your goal is to reach 150 pounds. So you go on some crazy diet and lose that 50 pounds. Great! You've reached your goal, but you haven't lowered your setpoint. In fact, because your body doesn't want to die of starvation, it has increased your setpoint to protect you in the future.

So in this theoretical scenario, if you ever stop starving yourself, it is a scientific fact that you will end up with more body fat than before. Michigan State University obesity researcher Dr. D. M. Garner confirms that "it is only the rate of weight regain, not the fact of weight regain, that appears open to debate" (Garner and Wooley 1991).

For an example of starvation's long-term side effects, consider a study by Leibel and Hirsch (1984) at Rockefeller University. A group of people weighing an average of 335 pounds starved themselves down to 220 pounds. After the starvation period was over, the researchers wanted to see what impact eating less had on the 220-pound dieters' need to burn body fat. To do this, they brought in people who were the same age but naturally weighed less. This gave the researchers three groups of people to compare:

1. Non-starved 335-pound people
2. Formerly 335-pound people who weighed 220 pounds
3. Non-starved 138-pound people

Like a larger SUV should need more gasoline than a smaller motorcycle, the non-starved 335-pound people should need more calories than the non-starved 138-pound people, right? Yes.

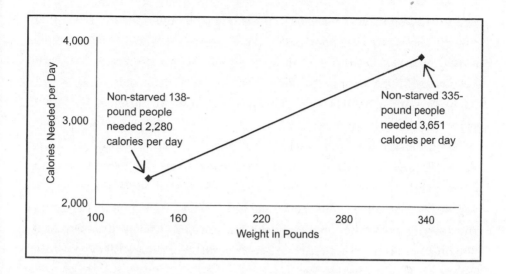

All things being equal, more body weight means more calories needed per day to maintain and move more mass. So after losing 115 pounds, you would think the 220-pound people must have slid down the graph and ended up here:

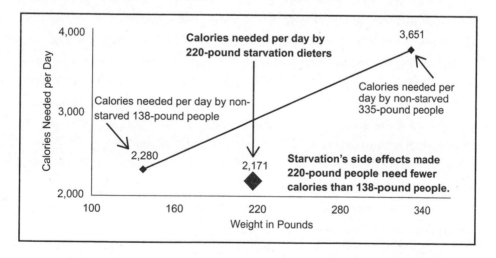

Right?

Not necessarily. It depends on how the 115 pounds were lost. After all, we know starvation burns calorie-hungry muscle while elevating your setpoint and slowing down your metabolism. So having starved away 115 pounds, how many calories did the 220-pound starvation dieters need?

Thanks to starvation's side effects, the 220-pound people destroyed their need to burn body fat. They ended up needing 5 percent fewer calories per day than the non-starved 138-pound people, even though they had 82 more pounds of mass to move. Let that sink in for a second. Starvation dieters who weigh 220 pounds MUST eat fewer calories than low-setpoint people who naturally weigh 138 pounds. That is why the harder we try to starve ourselves, the heavier we get.

Similar results were gained from a test done as far back as World War II. University of Minnesota researchers studied starvation to get a better understanding of how to help the hungry in war-torn Europe (Keys et al. 1950). The researchers recruited people in the United States and had them cut back to 1,600 calories per day.[1] Their metabolisms responded by slowing down by a whopping 40 percent. At the same time their strength fell by 28 percent, their endurance fell by 79 percent, and their rates of depression rose by 36 percent.

Let's focus on the metabolism slowing down by 40 percent for a moment. Say Jill needs and eats 2,000 calories per day. But now Jill wants to drop a few pounds for her vacation in 2 weeks, so she reads a magazine that tells her to starve herself, and she cuts back to 1,600 calories per day. According to this study, Jill's metabolism slows down by 40 percent and therefore she needs only 1,200 calories per day. Before Jill starved herself, she needed 2,000 calories per day and ate 2,000 calories per day. After starving herself, Jill only needed 1,200 calories per day but ate 1,600 per day. When she stops starving, she will eat 2,000 calories per day while only needing 1,200 calories per day. Then Jill's "hard work" will be rewarded with more weight than if she never bothered with dieting in the first place. Jill yo-yoed. Jill deserves better. And so do you!

You May Be Hormonally Clogged

If you've always had trouble losing weight and keeping it off, you may have a "hormonal clog," and it keeps your setpoint elevated.

When you become hormonally clogged, your body can no longer respond to signals from your hormones and brain that otherwise enable you to burn body fat automatically. However, when you increase the quality of your eating and exercise, you can heal your hormones, "unclog," lower your setpoint, and get your body to burn fat instead of store it.

---

[1] 1,600 calories per day is considered generous by today's "eat less" advocates.

An easy way to understand how this hormonal clog elevates your setpoint is to think about your body as being like a sink. When a sink is working properly, more water poured in means more water drains out. The water level may rise temporarily, but the sink will automatically take care of it. The sink is balancing water in and water out at a low level. The sink has a low setpoint.

A hormonally healthy body works similarly, doing its best to automatically keep excess fat from sticking around. A healthy body, like a "healthy" sink, responds to more in with more out, and to less in with less out. Water builds up in sinks, and fat builds up in bodies, only when they become clogged. The key question then is, What causes clogs?

Sinks and bodies get clogged and break down when the wrong *quality* of things are put in them. This is why you don't worry about washing your hands as quickly as possible, but you do work to keep hair out of your drain. You know that no *quantity* of the right quality will ever cause our sink to clog. Low quality, not high quantity, causes clogs.

Now, once clogs happen, any amount of water in will cause the water level to rise and stay high. You have a sink with an elevated setpoint. What do you do next?

You could use less water for the rest of your life, or you could use the same amount of water but spend an hour or two per day bailing excess water out of the sink. But why go through all that hassle when you could fix the underlying problem—by unclogging the sink (i.e., lowering your setpoint)?

Think of your body in the same way. When you put the wrong quality of food into it, your body becomes hormonally clogged, causing it to automatically balance you out at an elevated level of body fat. Like a backed-up sink with stagnant water sitting in it, you end up with a bunch of stagnant fat sitting in your body. These clogs can eventually lead to obesity, diabetes, and diabesity.

Once you're clogged and your body is balancing you at an elevated setpoint, you could cut calories and that would temporarily lower your weight. But why struggle through starvation? That's just like turning the faucet down. It doesn't actually fix anything, and it's tough to keep the faucet down forever.

So what should you do? How do you actually unclog your sink?

Very important: Focus on the *quality* of calories you put in your body, not the *quantity*. The truth is, calories work differently in the body depending on which food they come from.

As you will learn, the quality of calories varies wildly and is determined by four factors: Satiety, Aggression, Nutrition, and Efficiency (SANE).

> **S**atiety is how quickly calories fill you up.
> **A**ggression is how likely calories are to be stored as body fat.
> **N**utrition is how many vitamins, minerals, essential amino acids, essential fatty acids, and so forth, that calories provide.
> **E**fficiency is how easily calories are converted to body fat.

High-quality calories are Satisfying, unAggressive, Nutritious, and inEfficient. They include non-starchy vegetables, nutrient-dense proteins, whole-food fats, and low-fructose fruits. All of these foods are what I call SANE foods, which have transformational healing powers when it comes to clearing the biological "clogs" that elevate your setpoint. SANE foods trigger the release of body-fat-burning hormones, heal biological factors holding you back, and lower your setpoint. The more SANE foods you eat, the naturally slimmer you'll get.

You will absolutely love SANE foods, too, and you won't feel deprived. All your favorite tastes, flavors, and textures are part of a SANE lifestyle. And when it comes to quantity, the most common "complaint" I hear during this plan is, What if I am too full to eat all this food? Talk about "good problems"! As for cravings— like longing to bite into a glazed doughnut or getting up close and personal with a bag of chips—they'll disappear forever.

To illustrate the power of higher-quality SANE eating, consider a study from the University of Florida published in the *American Journal of Clinical Nutrition*, in which the researchers reviewed 87 studies and discovered that people who consumed higher-quality calories lost on average 12 more pounds of pure body fat, compared to dieters who ate the same number of calories but mostly from lower-quality, processed foods (Krieger et al. 2006). This study is great evidence that even without counting calories, a SANE diet full of non-starchy vegetables, nutrient-dense proteins, and whole-food fats produces lifesaving results.

There are hundreds of studies pointing to similar results regarding calorie quality versus calorie quantity. Long story short, some foods clog you and elevate your setpoint; others unclog you and lower your setpoint.

The evidence is the same for the treatment and management of diabetes. Harvard researchers reported in a 2014 issue of the *Lancet*: "The quality of dietary fats and carbohydrates consumed is more crucial than is the quantity of these macronutrients...to reduce the risk of diabetes and improve glycemic control and blood lipids in patients with diabetes" (Ley et al. 2014).

Now, how transformative is this information? You could close this book right now and have your life changed just by the knowledge that it's not about eating fewer calories but about improving the quality of the calories you eat. That distinction alone would change your health and life. Of course, more specifics on how to do this are coming, so don't put this book down just yet.

The bottom line is that by applying correct, science-backed principles, you can get wherever you want to go, no matter where you are right now. Instead of *struggling* to lose weight, you can repair your metabolism, lower your setpoint, and enjoy a body more like that of a naturally thin person. With a lower setpoint, naturally thin people are practically immune from weight gain. Their bodies burn excess calories and fat instead of storing them because they're "programmed" to stay at a low setpoint. Isn't it time you got to live that way, too?

I realize that everything we've covered here is likely totally different from what you've been told for decades. But isn't that *awesome*? I mean, if you want a totally different long-term result, doesn't it make sense to find that in a totally different approach? As Albert Einstein allegedly once said, the definition of insanity is "doing the same thing over and over and expecting different results." What if today was the day you stopped being tortured by the same starvation and shame-based nonsense over and over, being promised different results? What if you've finally discovered a totally different approach that gives you a totally different result?

You are about to find out.

SANE Points

- If you try to lose weight through starvation, you'll be condemned to an existence of perpetual yo-yo dieting, dissatisfaction with your appearance, increased health risks, and a constantly increasing setpoint.
- If you follow SANE principles, you can lower your setpoint and have a body that works more like the body of a naturally thin person. Without the frustration and deprivation of low-calorie diets, you can maintain your ideal weight loss long-term and leave behind the short-term fixes and soul-crushing yo-yo dieting.
- Calories count, but you don't need to count them. You need to select quality calories. They heal your body and brain and lower your setpoint. Then your brain will count calories for you like it did for every human who ever lived prior to anyone knowing about calories.
- Lowering your setpoint isn't just one way to lose weight; it's the only sustainable way to keep it off permanently.

CHAPTER 2

The Three Hidden Factors That Determine Your Weight

Lowering your setpoint is about healing your metabolism—not about being saturated with more and more shame. You know the pain and suffering associated with being overweight already. You are too important and valuable to be in such a constant state of misery. Please give yourself permission to stop trying to starve a disease—that you didn't cause—into submission.

It's time to do something very different to get a different result. With the SANE plan, you're on your way to healing a broken metabolism, lowering your setpoint, and steering clear of diets that make you heavier in the long run.

With the right nutritional and lifestyle choices, your body will work *with* you to keep weight off instead of fighting against you to keep weight on. The bottom line is that when you start eating and living SANEly, you will never think about weight loss or your body the same ever again. Once you realize that calorie-counting starvation diets actually increase your setpoint, everything will finally click, and you'll say, "Now I get why trying to lose weight in the past was so hard, and what I need to do instead to *permanently and enjoyably* reach my goals!"

Where we start is by looking at three primary factors that determine your setpoint: brain inflammation, gut bacteria, and hormones. Together these factors define and defend a range of about 20 pounds that your body fights to keep you within. When you understand these factors, you can begin to successfully lower your setpoint. You're now officially going down the road less traveled, and it will make all the difference. Get ready to meet the naturally thin you.

FACTOR #1: HEALTHY BRAIN, FLAT BELLY

What if healing your brain shrank your belly? While that may sound like science fiction, it's one of the little known scientific facts that will get you to your ideal setpoint and finally unlock permanent weight loss for you.

When you feel hungry, you probably think about your stomach. But did you know the feeling of hunger is all in your head? The link between your head and your stomach is the hypothalamus, an almond-sized structure located deep within your brain that serves a very vital function: the regulation and control of your metabolism. If the hypothalamus becomes "inflamed," your setpoint goes up, and you can have trouble staying at your ideal weight.

A little background: Inflammation is not necessarily a bad thing. It goes on throughout your body in various degrees and is essentially a vital part of the healing process. When you're injured or ill, your body wants to repair itself. Inflammation is part of this process. During inflammation, proteins called *cytokines* and fats with hormone-like properties called *prostaglandins* dilate blood vessels (vasodilation). This lets enzymes, antibodies, white blood cells, and nutrients access the injured area to fight infection and remove debris and bacteria.

Inflammation only turns into a problem if it continues for too long—in other words, becomes chronic. This can damage your organs and thus underlies many serious health problems: heart disease, diabetes, cancer, dementia, and, yes, obesity. Inflammation goes into overdrive for a variety of reasons such as poor nutrition, excessive stress, lack of sleep, and others.

But back to the hypothalamus: Researchers at the University of Washington and other institutions have discovered that an inflamed hypothalamus is one of the causes of overweight and obesity.

Dr. Michael Schwartz, a professor of medicine at the University of Washington, was the senior author of a paper titled "Obesity Is Associated with Hypothalamic Injury in Rodents and Humans," which was published in the *Journal of Clinical Investigation* in 2012. After humans and rodents ate an inSANE diet, their brains began to show evidence of inflammation in just 24 hours. If they kept eating inSANEly, the hypothalamus became seriously inflamed and showed structural damage.

His team also found that enjoying more SANE foods reduced inflammation in the brain. Those low-inflammation foods included those high in omega-3 fats such as salmon, flax seeds, and chia seeds.

The evidence linking brain inflammation to obesity has been building for some time. For example, a team of researchers from the University of Wisconsin School of Medicine and Public Health found that eating too many calories from sugary, high-fat inSANE foods definitely inflames the hypothalamus. This "neuroinflammation" then hijacks the normal operation of two key hormones, leptin and insulin. In a healthy body, these hormones act as messengers to regulate appetite and eating. But when they are disrupted, they can't effectively carry out their jobs. This leads to obesity, diabetes, and cardiovascular disease.

One more study underscores these findings. Italian scientists, publishing in *Frontiers in Cellular Neuroscience*, found that certain saturated fats such as lard are dangerous because—yes, you guessed it—they inflame the hypothalamus (Viggiano et al. 2016). Using two groups of rats, they observed that animals who were fed a diet high in saturated fat experienced a change in the hypothalamus that prevented them from regulating their food intake. Another group of rats was fed a similarly high-fat diet, but high in fish oil and not saturated fat. Those rats did not have any negative changes in their brain function. The researchers concluded that substituting unsaturated fats like fish oil, avocados, and olives could help reduce the risk for obesity in humans and possibly prevent other metabolic diseases.

Neuroinflammation also kills off neurons in other areas of the brain that are in charge of willpower. Willpower—wait a minute: Isn't that something we exert through sheer force of, well, will? No. When neurons are destroyed by neuroinflammation, certain brain chemicals become erratic and out of balance. Your brain goes into a "stimulus-seeking" mode that causes intense cravings. Regardless of your best intentions (willpower), you become consumed by a longing to devour sugary junk foods. However, when you eat SANEly, you will reverse neuroinflammation and be forever free from cravings.

Besides bad fats, other highly inflammatory foods are sugar, processed carbohydrates, and MSG (a food flavoring that breaks brain cells). By contrast, some of the most potent anti-inflammatory foods are high in omega-3 fats: highly colorful vegetables; low-fructose fruits; foods high in monounsaturated fats (e.g., macadamia nuts, cashews, avocados, olives); and to a lesser extent grass-fed beef, poultry, and eggs. On the 21-Day Plan and beyond, you'll focus on eating the most potently neurologically healing SANE foods.

The takeaway here is that we now have scientific proof for why sticking to traditional diets is so difficult—brain inflammation is sabotaging your efforts. Again, it's not an effort or character problem; it's a brain inflammation and medical problem.

FACTOR #2: YOUR OTHER BRAIN—THE GUT

Your body is composed of an estimated 100 trillion cells, but only about 10 percent are human. The rest are bacteria—up to 7 pounds' worth—and most of them are in the gut. This bacteria in your digestive system has a huge influence on your setpoint and your weight. Making up the "gut microbiota," these bacteria are responsible for a variety of tasks. They help extract calories from what you eat, store these calories for later use, and have a profound impact on whether you're overweight. Much of what we know comes from studies of rodents, but fear not, these little furry ones have helped us make some of the biggest breakthroughs in medical history, and they're doing the same for us here. Specifically, experiments on mice given gut bacteria from obese people showed they became fatter than those receiving microbes from lean people. In other words, transplanting the gut microbes from obese people fattened up the rodents.

The research into the effects of gut microbes on setpoint weight has been so compelling that it has birthed a related field of research around consuming pre- and probiotics to assist with weight loss. Reported in the *British Journal of Nutrition*, researchers at Laval University in Quebec found that probiotic supplements could help dieters lose weight and keep it off. Researchers recruited 125 overweight men and women. They followed a 12-week weight-loss diet, followed by a 12-week weight-loss maintenance period. Throughout the entire study, half the participants took daily two pills containing probiotics from the *Lactobacillus rhamnosus* family, while the other half received a placebo. The probiotic supplement also contained some prebiotics, which are dietary fibers on which probiotics feed.

After the 12-week diet period, the women in the probiotic group lost an average of nearly 10 pounds, while the placebo group lost about 5.5 pounds. (The probiotics didn't have any effect on the men.) But here's what's fascinating: After the 12-week maintenance period, the weight of the women in the placebo group remained stable, but the probiotic group continued to lose weight, for a total of more than 11 pounds per person! Bottom line, women taking probiotics lost twice as much weight over the 24-week study period (Sanchez, et al 2014).

Reported in the *European Journal of Clinical Nutrition*, an earlier study on probiotics conducted by Japanese researchers found that the probiotic *Lactobacillus gasseri* reduced belly fat, along with weight loss. During the study, researchers gave 87 overweight volunteers 100 grams of fermented milk, twice a day, with their normal diets. The milk drunk by half the group was enriched with the probiotic *L. gasseri*. After 12 weeks, these volunteers had lost an average of 2.2 pounds, while their counterparts showed no change in weight. Scans revealed that they had also lost 4.6 percent of their belly fat (Kadooka et al. 2010).

Remarkably, too, these tiny organisms play a big role by influencing the foods you crave. Research suggests that individual members of the microbiota have preferences for different types of food. For example, a gut microbe called *Prevotella* thrives best on carbohydrates, *Bifidobacterium* likes dietary fiber, and Bacteroidetes prefer to feast on certain fats. A 2007 study published in the *Journal of Proteome Research* found that people who are "chocolate desiring" have different microbial metabolites in their urine than "chocolate indifferent" individuals (Rezzi et al. 2007). So the next time you feel an irresistible craving for sweets, *again*, it is not due to a lack of self-control; it is because that's what your not-yet-SANEitized gut bugs are craving.

The big takeaway here is: If you want to enlist billions of microscopic setpoint-lowering bacterial minions into your campaign against weight gain, do not starve yourself or eat processed prepackaged diet food. Both of those tactics kill the little guys you need on your side. Instead, eat so much setpoint-lowering SANE food that you are too full for inSANE, setpoint-elevating products. This feeds the gut bacterial minions you need to succeed while helping to eliminate the little bacterial buggers who drive your setpoint up.

FACTOR #3: HORMONES: THE BRIDGE BETWEEN BOTH BRAINS

You can't hear it or see it, but there's a whole lot of chitchat going on inside you all the time. Your gut, organs, muscle tissue, and fat tissue are constantly communicating with your nervous system and brain via chemical messengers called *hormones*. They "talk" about, for example, how much fuel they think you need to keep your weight stable at your setpoint. If they feel you're at risk of your weight falling below your setpoint, they relay chemical messages that drive your appetite and cravings up and your daily calorie burn down.

When you eat high-quality calories, this conversation goes well. Higher-quality calories trigger fat-burning hormones. The right amount of hormones are used and the desired message is communicated: "Burn body fat."

However, when you eat low-quality, processed calories, it's like the phone lines break down. Your body doesn't have a good idea of how much fuel you need. Hormones become "dysregulated," and your body demands more food and hoards calories, because it does not know what is going on and errs on the side of not starving. Remember the analogy of the clogged sink? This is how that "hormonal clog" I talked about earlier gets created.

This clog elevates your setpoint and therefore triggers a 24/7/365 increase in appetite and cravings and a decrease in energy and calorie burn. More calories in and less calories out is what just about every cell in your body is telling you to do to survive. Even if you do grit your teeth and stick to your starvation diet and daily jog, this "hormonal clog" will cause your body to store more of the calories you eat as fat, while burning fewer off during exercise. In other words, you do what the "boot camp" instructor tells you, you "try harder," but basic human biology causes your body to fight back by storing more and burning less.

As you can see, hormones play a huge role in regulating your setpoint. Fortunately, you aren't at their mercy. There's a lot you can do to control your hormones and how they influence calories in, calories out, and setpoint. You just have to understand what they are and how they work. There are several main hormones that impact your setpoint and how well your body burns fat.

Leptin

Your fat cells produce a hormone called *leptin*, which signals your brain when it's had enough food. As fat stores rise, more leptin is secreted, traveling to the brain with the message "Your levels of body fat are on the rise so I'm going to make you feel full and fidgety so you unconsciously 'eat less and exercise more.'" If fat levels fall, so do leptin levels, and your brain gets a strong hormonal signal to eat more and burn less. Leptin drives your motivation to eat and move, not willpower.

Before you are victimized by Internet ads for leptin supplements, please understand: Overweight people already have lots of leptin (remember, it's secreted in proportion to the amount of fat on your body). The problem is, your setpoint gets elevated when you suffer from "leptin resistance," in which the hormone is unable to get its message across. Therefore, increasing leptin levels to treat an elevated setpoint is as productive as adding water to a fish tank with no bottom.

You can ensure that leptin gets the job done by healing the metabolic breakdowns causing "leptin resistance." Guess what makes the metabolic breakdowns worse? Conventional low-calorie high-carb starvation diets. Guess what solves the problem? Exactly what you'll do on the 21-Day Plan. Woohoo!

Ghrelin

This hormone is all about appetite. Remember that when you cut calories and undereat, your body revolts. It starts defending a higher setpoint. As part of this defense, your brain signals an increase in ghrelin to get you to eat more. With traditional starvation diets, ghrelin increases. This is another big reason why traditional diets have failed you. They only make you hungrier and tell you to eat foods that caused the hormonal clog in the first place! Again, "you" are not doing anything "wrong." Rather, ghrelin is out of balance, and you'll be taking the right measures to get it back in check.

Insulin

We can't talk about fat-burning hormones without talking about insulin, which is produced in the pancreas. For glucose to get into cells to be burned for fuel, it needs open "doors" to the cells. These doors are the insulin receptors on the cells' surfaces. Insulin's function is to usher glucose into cells through those receptors.

When your body digests the sugars and starches you eat, it breaks them down into glucose, which gets absorbed into the bloodstream. Your insulin automatically spikes to shuttle the glucose into cells. If you eat too much sugary, starchy, highly processed food (inSANE calories), glucose levels stay elevated longer than they need to. More insulin is cranked out, and it has to work overtime. When insulin is elevated 24/7, insulin receptors on cells get so used to it that they stop recognizing it—a condition known as *insulin resistance*. Think of this situation like stuck doors; they (the cell receptors) just won't open.

Insulin must still do its job of removing glucose from the bloodstream, however, so when most of the cells in the body won't "open up" to it, the insulin has no choice but to take the glucose somewhere else: to your fat cells. Fat cells will *always* accept more energy for storage. This initiates the vicious cycle of high insulin, high blood glucose levels, and, of course, more fat storage. If this cycle continues long enough, all the non-fat cells in your body scream, "We are starving!" This causes the body to respond by increasing its setpoint. In the wake of this increase comes obesity, insulin resistance, prediabetes, type 2 diabetes, and diabesity. Therefore, keeping insulin levels in check is vital not just for preventing diabetes, but also for maintaining a healthy, low setpoint and weight.

It's also about more than simply shedding pounds. Insulin plays a key role in *where* body fat gets stored. Lots of insulin hanging around for long periods of time creates more abdominal fat—not so fondly referred to as a "menopot" for millions of women over the age of 40. This amplifies your risk for a variety of serious illnesses, including type 2 diabetes, diabesity, and heart disease.

To achieve your ideal setpoint, you have to lower insulin levels. You'll learn how to do this naturally, automatically, and deliciously by eating SANE foods.

Testosterone

This hormone is commonly thought of as a male hormone, but both men and women need adequate testosterone levels to keep their setpoint low. Most adult women have about the same testosterone levels as a 10-year-old boy. That's part of the reason it is harder for women to burn fat and build muscle than it is for men. Low levels of testosterone promote fat storage and inflammation. Excess testosterone in women, especially around menopause, is associated with insulin resistance and belly fat. You can see why having this hormone in the right balance is so important.

Eating lots of refined carbohydrates and soy foods will downshift testosterone and elevate setpoint, in both men and women. On the other hand, nutrient-dense proteins and whole-food fats as well as "eccentric" exercise (which you'll read about later) optimizes testosterone, lowering your setpoint.

Estrogen

Like testosterone, estrogen is present in both men and women, though is higher in women. A few years prior to menopause, however, a woman's estrogen levels begin to dip—which makes her body hold on to fat. The good news is that the same nutrition and lifestyle factors that optimize testosterone levels to favor a lower setpoint also shift estrogen in better balance for both women and men. More coming, but from a high level, replacing starches and sweets with SANE veggies, proteins, and fats, plus SANE lifestyle upgrades around exercise, sleep, and stress, optimize estrogen.

Stress Hormones

Secreted by the adrenal glands, stress hormones are involved in weight and hunger signals. One of the most influential on setpoint and weight is cortisol.

Among cortisol's many functions is to trigger the release of insulin to get glucose into cells for the energy to deal with short-term stress. This is a part of your body's survival response to stress. If a tiger starts chasing you (the typical type of short-term stress humans faced for the majority of our history), you need fuel fast. Then the crisis ends, the glucose is burned off, and a relaxation response gradually returns the body's systems to normal.

This is a normal and lifesaving response from your body. The trouble is that your body responds to *all* stresses in the same way. If you are experiencing marital problems, financial worries, job stress, starvation, or worry, guilt, and shame over your weight, it's all "a tiger is chasing you right now" from your body's perspective.

This is not good because these chronic sources of stress cause your body to keep churning out cortisol as if you were *always* right on the verge of becoming a tiger snack. Because cortisol prompts the release of insulin, that hormone stays elevated, too, and based on what you just learned about insulin, this is all sorts of bad. But we're not done yet because unlike physical stress, psychological stress does not burn off glucose, so now we've got a setpoint-elevating trifecta of constantly elevated cortisol, insulin, and glucose!

But wait, there's more. The insulin resistance caused by this cortisol chaos triggers feedback to the brain indicating that cells aren't getting glucose, which then leads to cravings for more glucose. Guess where you find the most glucose? Sugar and starches. Know what makes weight loss nearly impossible? Intense sugar and starch cravings. Also, now you know why when you get stressed, the comfort food craved always revolves around sugar and starch. Why? Your brain "thinks" it needs glucose to prevent a tiger from tearing you in half, so you end up tearing a bag of potato chips in half for your own survival.

In short, chronically elevated cortisol leads to increased insulin, insulin resistance, sugar and starch cravings, even more insulin, even more intense cravings, an elevated setpoint, weight gain, prediabetes, and then type 2 diabetes. It's a vicious cycle, but we're still not done. Fat cells "in" your belly (visceral fat) have a large number of receptors for cortisol—so all that fat from chronic psychological stress is preferentially put right on your belly. All of that makes you feel bad about yourself (body shame), which causes more stress. That compounds cravings for sugar and starches, which goes right back and makes all of those things worse. It's a catastrophic cortisol cascade of chaos that partly explains why one in four middle-age women are prescribed antidepressants—what else are we supposed to do in a *seemingly* hopeless trap like this? I get it. And I promise that we can do better for you. It gets better…and we'll do it together.

Thyroid Hormones

We could very easily spend all of our time on only hormones, but we need to get to the solution to all of this, so let's pick up the pace.

Restrictive, starvation-type dieting slows the function of your thyroid and your metabolism, thus elevating your setpoint. The thyroid produces the thyroid hormones: an inactive form called *thyroxine* (T4) and an active form called *triiodothyronine* (T3). The T4 is transported through the blood, and once it reaches each cell, it is converted to the active T3 form.

Both hormones regulate your metabolism, which, in turn, impacts your setpoint along with your heart, brain, digestion, and other bodily systems. So if your thyroid isn't rocking and rolling, it can affect almost every aspect of your health.

The most common problem is an underactive thyroid, or hypothyroidism, where levels of thyroid hormone are less than optimal. Among the main symptoms are fatigue, feeling cold, dry skin, weight gain (about 5 to 20 pounds), insulin resistance, depression, hair loss, and memory problems. More women than men suffer from hypothyroidism, largely due to fluctuating hormones during various life changes: onset of puberty, during and after pregnancy, at or just before menopause, and during postmenopause.

Other Setpoint Hormones

Cholecystokinin (CCK) is involved in satiety. Research has found that overeating can make receptors on cells less sensitive to CCK. This triggers another vicious cycle: The more low-quality food you eat, the less your body recognizes the signal to slow down. Thankfully, you are "going SANE" and will eat so much high-quality food that you'll have no room for CCK "slowing" inSANE food.

Next is adiponectin. Secreted by fat cells, this helps regulate blood sugar and promotes fat-burning. In combination with leptin, it reverses insulin resistance. Levels stabilize when you lower your setpoint, replace starches and sweets with non-starchy veggies, and nutrient-dense proteins, and improve your fitness.

As you clear your hormonal clogs through SANE eating and living, your setpoint will fall, and you will experience something you may have thought was impossible: eating as much as you want, whenever you want, while easily maintaining an ideal weight. Why? Because that's what your hormones tell your body to do, and that's what SANE eating and living tells your hormones to do. Always. For everyone.

OTHER FACTORS THAT AFFECT YOUR SETPOINT

Although we're going to spend a majority of our time talking about setpoint-lowering nutrition, exercise, psychology, and lifestyle habits, you're also going to learn about other factors that add just the right kick to lower your setpoint and keep it there for life. In fact, practically every choice you make affects your setpoint to some degree.

Take a look at the SANE Setpoint Lifestyle Spectrum below. The more SANE a choice is, the more it lowers your setpoint; the more inSANE a choice is, the more it increases your setpoint.

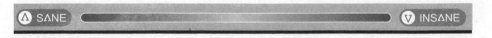

Extreme Setpoint Decrease	Major Setpoint Decrease	Minor Setpoint Decrease	No Impact	Minor Setpoint Increase	Major Setpoint Increase	Extreme Setpoint Increase
8 hours a night of quality sleep	Smarter exercise	Sweating	Almost nothing (every choice you make impacts your setpoint)	Improper exercise and too much of it	SSRIs	Starvation dieting
10 servings of non-starchy veggies	Meditation	Stove vs. microwave		Toxins in food	Starchy, sugary foods	Stress
Balanced testosterone/ estrogen	SANE nutraceuticals	Organic foods		Sitting		Sodas
SANE green smoothies	SANE superfoods	Standing		Processed "nutrition" bars	The news	Shame
Loving relationships	Healthy sex life	Smiling			Diet pills	Unbalanced insulin/ cortisol

While we can't cover everything that impacts your setpoint in this chapter, this is where the Web works wonders. You can get more information on how everything you can think of (and even some things you can't think of) impacts your setpoint at SANESolution.com. For now, let's stay focused on the big things that give you the best results with the least effort: SANE eating, SANE movement, and SANE psychology. You'll see how it comes together once the 21-Day Plan begins. More than 1,300 studies and tens of thousands of success stories are on your side. If you want to reprogram your body to behave like a naturally thin person, you're about to make that happen, easily and effortlessly—and experience dramatically better health and astonishing results.

SANE Points

- The three primary factors that determine your setpoint are brain inflammation, gut bacteria, and hormone levels. Heal these factors with SANE nutrition and SANE living, and you lower your setpoint and therefore weight automatically. No willpower necessary.
- A SANE lifestyle with the right nutrition, smart activity, good-quality sleep, and low levels of unhealthy stress will lower your setpoint, help you drop pounds, and maintain a slim life like that of a naturally thin person.
- Live on the SANE side of the SANE spectrum, and you'll maintain a low setpoint permanently.

PART 2

SANE FOODS

CHAPTER 3

Good Calories, Bad Calories, and SANE Calories...Oh My!

Think for a moment about people who are naturally thin. How do they get that way? They eat whatever they want, they don't really exercise, and they still stay slim. What does a body of a naturally thin person do that enables it to be thin, effortlessly and permanently? More importantly, what can *you* do so that your body acts like the body of a naturally thin person?

We've already answered that: lower your setpoint. While naturally thin people were lucky enough to be born that way, with this plan, you can live the rest of your life that way. The best place to start is by eating more SANE food. Far from eating less, you will be eating *more* food than you ever have in your life...from SANE sources. In fact, one of the most common questions our coaches get is, What if I'm too full to eat all of this food? Not a bad problem to have while losing weight!

SANE foods all hinge around "calorie quality." Remember, calories work differently in the body, depending on which food they come from. Putting 1,000 calories of low-quality food (think chips and soda) into your body has radically different effects on your weight than ingesting the same quantity of high-quality calories (think salmon and avocados). The more low-quality inSANE calories you eat, the higher your setpoint.[2] The more high-quality SANE calories you eat, the lower your setpoint.

---

[2] This explains why starvation diets DO cause weight loss in the short term. Since about 50 percent of the typical diet comes from inSANE low-quality calories, eating less of that diet will cause

The quality of calories is determined by four factors: **S**atiety, **A**ggression, **N**utrition, and **E**fficiency. The "SANE" approach to eating considers them all. SANE will change the way you think about food, calories, and even yourself.

You are high quality, and you deserve high-quality calories. Let's be honest, we're talking about putting food inside you. And we're talking about what food is being put inside our children and loved ones. I think it's worth the effort to ensure only high-quality products are being put inside ourselves and those we love. Here's how you do that.

CALORIE QUALITY #1: SATIETY

Are you tired of being hungry and tired? If so, one word can change your life: *Satiety*. It's how scientists measure how "satisfying" various foods are. For example, a food with high Satiety satisfies you quickly and keeps you satisfied for a long time. On the other hand, foods like Pringles (aka "once you pop, you can't stop") have low Satiety because you must eat a lot of them to feel satisfied—and even then, it doesn't last long.

If you want to easily avoid hunger AND overeating, eat more high-Satiety foods in place of low-Satiety foods. For example, eat more meatballs, and you will have less room for the pasta. The more high-Satiety foods you eat, the fuller you are, making it harder to eat setpoint-increasing foods. By eating more of the "right" things, you effortlessly avoid the "wrong" things. It's the simple and powerful science of Satiety. It makes willpower obsolete—and that changes everything.

I'm not suggesting you never eat sweets. I'm only asking you to imagine how your life would be different if you were always so full and satisfied that cravings for sweets went away. It can happen—I see it every day.

The fewer calories needed to fill you up (and the longer those calories keep you full), the higher the satiety of that food. And you won't be hungry because high-Satiety calories are also the most Nutritious calories in the world (the **S** and **N** in SANE), so it's a win-win. No points or calorie counting needed. Your beautiful biology does that for you.

---

weight loss, but only until you get sick and tired of being sick and tired thanks to disordered eating and starvation dieting.

All sorts of research shows that calorie for calorie, certain foods are more filling than others. A study published in the *Annals of Internal Medicine* followed 10 obese patients with type 2 diabetes for 21 days, and found that the people who ate as much high-Satiety protein and natural fat as they wanted, while avoiding low-Satiety starches and sweets, unconsciously avoided *1,000 low-quality calories per day* (Boden et al. 2005). And these participants reported feeling just as satisfied as other people in the study who ate 1,000 *more* lower-Satiety calories.

Why is eating 1,000 fewer low-quality calories per day useful? Didn't we just cover how harmful starvation is? Yes, but we're not talking starvation here. When you eat high-Satiety food, you take in more food and much more nutrition, but unintentionally get full faster, stay full longer, and therefore automatically avoid overeating. More food, more nutrition, more energy, and unconsciously avoiding excessive calories is entirely different from less food, less nutrition, feeling hungry, and being tired and cranky all day. The surplus of nutrition and satisfaction from high-satiety food saves you from the side effects of starvation.

The primary area in your brain influenced by high-Satiety foods is the hypothalamus. It tells you when you feel satisfied from eating. Its "you are satisfied" signals that tell you to stop eating depend on three factors:

1. How much do the calories you're eating stretch your digestive organs?
2. How much do the calories you're eating affect short-term Satiety hormones?
3. How much do the calories you're eating stimulate long-term Satiety hormones?

You can enjoy more high-Satiety food by focusing on foods that contain high amounts of water, fiber, and protein. How much a food stretches your stomach and other digestive organs is mostly determined by the amount of water and fiber in it. More water and fiber mean bigger food, more stretch, and getting fuller and staying fuller longer. That is why 200 calories of wet, fibrous celery is more filling than 200 calories of dry, fiber-free gummy bears. Calorie for calorie, celery is about 30 times the size of gummy bears, stretches your stomach and other digestive organs much more, and is therefore much more satisfying.

Foods high in water include non-starchy vegetables, low-fructose fruits, and (surprise) nutrient-dense protein,[3] all of which help to fill you up. Noted researchers like Barbara Rolls at Pennsylvania State University and Adam Drewnowski at the University of Washington have published extensive science demonstrating that feeling full is linked to the size and weight (i.e., volume) of foods. In fact, Dr. Rolls has referred to water in foods as "the secret ingredient" to Satiety.

Dietary fiber is another "secret" ingredient. Unlike other food components such as fats, proteins, or carbohydrates—which your body breaks down and absorbs—fiber isn't digested by your body. Taking up space in your digestive system until it "makes you regular," fiber keeps you full for a long time.

The amount of protein in food is also critical. Publishing in the *Journal of the American College of Nutrition*, Harvard researchers have found that protein affects the other two factors that influence your "stop eating" and "say full" signals: short- and long-term satiety hormones. More calories from protein mean more "full" hormonal signals being sent to your brain now and later (Halton and Hu 2004).

Short-term satiety hormones include ghrelin, which initiates the feeling of hunger, and another hormone called peptide tyrosine tyrosine (PYY). Produced by gut cells and released into the bloodstream, PYY travels to the brain to decrease hunger and boost satiety. This slows the movement of food in the gut, thereby ensuring maximum digestion of nutrients and decreased appetite.

Long-term satiety hormones include leptin and insulin, both triggered by eating. Produced by fat cells, leptin sends "I'm full" signals to your brain. Protein keeps levels of glucose-managing insulin in check for long periods of time so that your blood sugar doesn't dip, leaving you hungry.

The power of protein to tame appetite and promote feelings of fullness has been shown repeatedly in numerous clinical trials:

- In a University of Washington study, participants ate an unlimited quantity of calories while having the proportion of protein in their diet increased from 15 percent to 30 percent. They responded by unconsciously avoiding 441 excess calories per day without feeling hungry (Boden et al. 2005).

---

[3] Fish and meat are high in water? Thirsty…Eat a steak? Yes…sort of. Look no further than jerky. Beef, turkey, and salmon jerky are those foods with the water removed. Beef, turkey, and salmon are mostly water by weight, and that's why their jerky brethren are so much smaller and lighter.

- In a University of Sussex study, participants ate either a high-protein or a low-protein meal. The high-protein people unconsciously ate 26 percent less than the low-protein people at their next meal without feeling hungry (Booth et al. 1970).
- In a University of Leeds study, participants ate the exact same weight of food, but one group ate a higher percent from protein. The higher-protein group unconsciously ate at least 19 percent fewer calories than the lower-protein group without feeling hungry (Hill and Blundell 1986).
- In a Karolinska Hospital study, participants ate more or less protein for lunch. The more-protein group got full on 12 percent fewer calories at dinner than the less-protein group (Barkeling et al. 1990).

The science is clear: More water, fiber, and protein mean more Satiety. More Satiety means you can get too full for setpoint-raising, low-quality food. Bottom line: High-Satiety eating makes high-willpower living unnecessary. (And that's awesome!)

CALORIE QUALITY #2: AGGRESSION

There's an old saying that goes like this: "Two minutes on your lips, a lifetime on your hips."

The problem with this statement is that "2 minutes" may or may not end up on your hips, or anywhere else on your body for that matter. The reason is that calories vary in how likely they are to be stored as body fat. The more Aggressive calories are, the more your body will store them as fat.

What makes calories Aggressive? In a nutshell: how quickly they flood your body with glucose. Your body can handle a sharp spike in glucose every once in a while. But constantly elevated glucose levels give your body no choice but to use fat tissue as the preferred depot for that glucose (this literally turns your body into a body fat–creating machine). The more sugar and starch—and the less fiber, protein, and fat—in a food, the more Aggressive it is (bad) and the more likely its calories are to be shuttled into fat storage.

Examples of Aggressive calories are sweets and starches. Suppose you eat a big plate of pasta, along with some garlic bread (starch plus starch). Dessert is a few cookies (starch plus sugar). Those calories are so Aggressive that your body will send them right into fat storage.

Anytime the body has more starchy and sugary calories available than it can deal with at one time, it stores them as body fat. That is why the *glycemic index* and *glycemic load* have become so well known in nutrition. *Glycemic index* refers to a measure of a food's Aggression—how high it spikes your blood sugar. The higher a food's glycemic index, the more Aggressive it is. Glycemic load is similar to glycemic index but also considers quantity. The glycemic load measures a food's Aggression combined with the carbohydrates in a portion of it.

Bottom line: Your body will drive the fat storage process when you have more glucose in your bloodstream than your body can use at one time. The more Aggressive calories are, the faster they increase the levels of glucose in your bloodstream and the faster those calories head to fat cells.

Fortunately, you don't have to worry about memorizing the glycemic index or glycemic load of foods because SANE eating prevents excess glucose from getting into your bloodstream. When you stick to increasing the amount of water-, fiber-, and protein-packed high-Satiety foods, you automatically eat low-glycemic foods, ensure a low-glycemic load, and store less body fat. You also lower your risk of diabetes, unhealthy cholesterol levels, and cardiovascular disease.

What about fat? You do not have to worry about fat in whole foods being Aggressive. Eating fat does not increase the amount of glucose in your bloodstream at all. In fact, digesting fat slows the release of glucose into the bloodstream. That is why foods containing fat are often less Aggressive than fat-free foods, and a lot of those "low-fat" products you see touted are actually more Aggressive because they are making up for the lack of fat with added sugars. That said, foods made up of nothing but fat—like oils, butter, and cream—are not SANE because they don't contain any water, fiber, and very little protein. They are fine if absolutely needed when cooking, but your setpoint would be lower if you ate fats in whole-food form instead.

CALORIE QUALITY #3: NUTRITION

What if everything you were taught about nutrition was wrong? I've got good news and bad news. The good news is that it's not *all* wrong. The bad news is that it's incomplete. But there is one more bit of good news: With three simple words—*nutrients per calorie*—you can see the real world of nutrition and your set-point will never be the same.

When you look at the nutritional breakdown on food labels, you may look at the calorie count and then all the details below it. All good. You are halfway there. The only thing left to unlock a whole new world of setpoint-lowering nutrition is to divide those details by the number of calories. Wait—on second thought, you don't actually have to do any algebra. You just need to keep in mind that anything that anyone says about nutrition that isn't framed in terms of "per calorie" is at best incomplete and at worst wrong.

This is true because *nutrition* refers to the vitamins, minerals, essential amino acids, essential fatty acids, fiber, antioxidants, and phytonutrients (beneficial plant chemicals) found in food. However, the number of calories found in foods varies wildly, so talking about the nutrition of a food without considering the calories within that food is like talking about parenting without considering the age of the child. For instance, which is more nutritious, a cup of enriched wheat flour or a cup of spinach? Ignoring calories and just comparing the other details on the labels you would see:

Nutrients per Cup

Nutrients	Enriched Wheat Flour (% DV)	Spinach (% DV)
Vitamin A	0	56
Vitamin C	0	14
Vitamin E	3	3
Vitamin K	1	181
Thiamine	74	2
Riboflavin	41	3
Niacin	52	1
Vitamin B6	3	3
Folate	63	15
Calcium	2	3
Iron	34	5

Nutrients	Enriched Wheat Flour (% DV)	Spinach (% DV)
Magnesium	9	6
Phosphorus	13	1
Potassium	4	5
Zinc	8	1

DV: Recommended Daily Value based on a 2,000-calorie diet.

If you stopped there, enriched wheat flour appears to be more nutritious overall. And that's why the USDA's various pyramids and plates continue to tell us grains are nutritious. Here's why that's objectively wrong. One cup of enriched wheat flour contains 495 calories. One cup of spinach contains 7 calories. Does it seem fair or even logical to compare 495 calories of one food to 7 calories of another food? No way! To be fair, scientifically accurate, and to lower your setpoint, you can fix this by looking at nutrients per calorie. For example, here's how the nutrition of enriched wheat flour and spinach compare if you look at nutrient per calorie:

Nutrients per 250 Calories

Nutrients	Enriched Wheat Flour (% DV)	Spinach (% DV)
Vitamin A	0	2,000
Vitamin C	0	500
Vitamin E	2	107
Vitamin K	1	6,464
Thiamine	37	71
Riboflavin	21	107
Niacin	26	36
Vitamin B6	2	107
Folate	32	536
Calcium	1	107
Iron	17	179

Nutrients	Enriched Wheat Flour (% DV)	Spinach (% DV)
Magnesium	5	214
Phosphorus	7	36
Potassium	2	179
Zinc	4	36

When you look at those magic three words—*nutrients per calorie*—you get a whole new and super slimming view of Nutrition. It's really cool and leads to food guide pyramids and plates that look like these:[4]

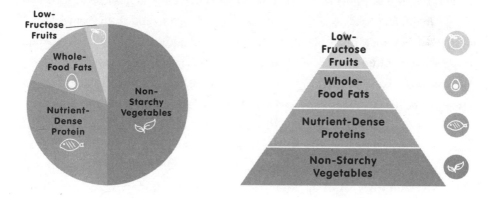

So, in your new world of SANEity, *Nutrition* with a capital *N* (aka the *N* in SANE) means "nutrients per calorie." That distinction gives you a more accurate view of food, and more importantly, it will save your life. Basically, the more nutrients (vitamins, minerals, essential proteins, essential fats, etc.) concentrated into a food calorie, the more beneficial it is. The fewer nutrients per calorie, the less healthy and more setpoint-elevating it is.

As we alluded to when discussing Satiety and Aggression, Nutrition plays a big part in lowering your setpoint. When you eat more water-, fiber-, and protein-filled foods, you get more essential nutrients while avoiding overeating (Satiety) or overwhelming the body with glucose (Aggression). A University of Florida study discovered that people who ate more nutrient-dense foods enjoyed lower levels of body fat and inflammation than people who ate the exact same number of calories, but

---

[4] These factor in that protein and fat are essential while sugar is not. More on that later.

from foods that were not nutrient dense (Kadey 2015). A surplus of quality nutrition is the opposite of starvation and your key to fat loss instead of frustration.

Maximizing Nutrition is easy: simply choose foods high in water, protein, and fiber. These include non-starchy vegetables; low-fructose fruits like berries; nuts, seeds, and other whole fats; and quality proteins like humanely raised fish and meat.

WHAT ABOUT "HEALTHY" WHOLE GRAINS?

Aren't "healthy whole grains" the foundation of any good diet? Sadly, no. Just because some food products are "whole grain" doesn't mean they're SANE—for several reasons. They don't fill you up when compared calorie for calorie to veggies and protein (**S**atiety). They make glucose levels skyrocket (which leads to fat storage—**A**ggression). They contain fewer nutrients than their non-starchy plant-food counterparts (**N**utrition), and they are in**E**fficient (which I'll get to in a moment). You don't need grains to lower your setpoint and optimize health. Further, if you eat grains *instead of* SANEr foods like non-starchy veggies, nutrient-dense protein, whole-food fats, and low-fructose fruits, you are increasing your setpoint and harming your health.

Is whole-wheat toast SANEr than a doughnut? Yes. But that's not saying much. Is one pack of cigarettes "healthier" than two? Yes! But again, something being "less bad" is not the same as it being awesome at lowering your setpoint. Whole grains are "less bad" than what makes up most diets. That doesn't mean they are good for you. And it definitely does not mean they are an effective way to lower your setpoint.

For example, take a look at how 1 cup of whole-wheat pasta stacks up against 1 cup of zucchini noodles or "zoodles" (a SANE food many of our members are deliciously substituting for pasta) in terms of nutrient quality.

Nutrients per Cup

Nutrients	Whole-Wheat Pasta (Cooked) (% DV)	Zoodles (Cooked) (% DV)
Calories	174 calories	8 calories
Dietary fiber	25	8
Vitamin A	0	12
Vitamin B6	9	12
Vitamin B12	0	0
Thiamine	11	5

Nutrients	Whole-Wheat Pasta (Cooked) (% DV)	Zoodles (Cooked) (% DV)
Riboflavin	4	3
Niacin	5	5
Folate	2	13
Vitamin C	0	39
Vitamin D	0	0
Vitamin E	3	2
Vitamin K	1	7
Calcium	3	4
Potassium	14	87
Iron	19	9
Magnesium	12	10
Phosphorus	13	7
Copper	12	5
Manganese	97	16
Zinc	8	4

DV: Recommended daily value based on a 2,000-calorie diet.

Looking at quantity, whole-wheat pasta seems more nutritious than zoodles in nutrients such as fiber, thiamine, and several minerals (iron, magnesium, phosphorous, copper, manganese, selenium, and zinc). But here's why that's misleading: 1 cup of whole-wheat pasta contains 174 calories, and 1 cup of zoodles contains 27 calories. But looking at quality—nutrients per calorie—you see something much different and more useful. Here is a more fair comparison—comparing 174 calories of pasta to 27 calories of zoodles:

Nutrients per Cup

Nutrients	Whole-Wheat Pasta (Cooked) (% DV)	Zoodles (Cooked) (% DV)
Calories	8 (174 cals.)	1 (27 cals.)
Dietary fiber	25	52
Vitamin A	0	77
Vitamin B6	9	77
Vitamin B12	0	0

Nutrients	Whole-Wheat Pasta (Cooked) (% DV)	Zoodles (Cooked) (% DV)
Thiamine	11	32
Riboflavin	4	19
Niacin	5	32
Folate	2	84
Vitamin C	0	251
Vitamin D	0	0
Vitamin E	3	13
Vitamin K	1	45
Calcium	3	26
Potassium	14	561
Iron	19	58
Magnesium	12	65
Phosphorus	13	45
Copper	12	32
Manganese	97	103
Zinc	8	26

DV: Recommended daily value based on a 2,000-calorie diet.

Knowing these facts, why would any nutritionist tell you to eat more whole-wheat pasta instead of telling you to eat more zoodles? I mean heck, "zoodles" is even more fun to say!

Like Satiety and Aggression, a food's Nutrition depends on water, fiber, and protein. Water and fiber have no calories, and protein calories do not "count" as much as carbohydrate or fat calories (more on this when we talk about Efficiency…the *E* in SANE). When you keep water, fiber, and protein at the top of your mind, you'll have a dramatically different view of which foods are nutritious.

Let me pick on grains again only because when I was growing up, the Food Guide Pyramid convinced me that they were the most nutritious foods in the world. Consider cereal, bread, rice, pasta, or all the other "healthy" starches sitting in most pantries. The reason they are in the pantry and not the fridge or freezer is because they contain no water. Strike one. They also contain little protein.[5] Strike two. Fiber is their only hope.

---

[5] This includes the trendy grain quinoa. For example, say you want more protein in your lunch and can choose between quinoa salad and tuna salad. Calorie for calorie, tuna contains six times

But be cautious about the high-fiber claims companies make for their whole-grain products. Are they actually true? The 4 grams of fiber in 250 calories of whole-grain cereal *is* double the fiber in 2 grams of fiber in 250 calories of refined-grain cereal, but that is only comparing grains. We have to ask if grains are a good source of fiber compared with more water- and protein-packed foods you could be eating. Spoiler alert: They are not. Eating whole-grain bread to get more fiber is like eating carrot cake to get more vegetables.

To wrap up, it's a good thing you are already focusing on foods rich in water, fiber, and protein when it comes to Satiety and Aggression because those are the same three factors that give you REAL setpoint-lowering Nutrition.

CALORIE QUALITY #4: EFFICIENCY

The fourth and final part of the SANE acronym might be the most revolutionary and is definitely the least well known in the mainstream. The *E* in SANE stands for "Efficiency." Your body varies wildly in its ability to store things you consume as body fat. Some things you consume can't be stored as fat, while others are very Efficiently stored as body fat. If your goal is having less fat on your body, it's helpful to eat foods that your body is inEfficient at storing as body fat.

Before you can identify which foods are Efficiently stored as body fat (and then avoid them), you need a bit of background on how your body handles food in general. From a volume perspective, food is made up of essentially fiber, water, protein, carbohydrate/sugar/starch, and fat. Fiber and water don't provide your body with calories, so they are not applicable here. You could say that fiber, water, or anything else that your body can't get calories from is 100 percent inEfficient. That means you could consume it in unlimited quantities and never store any of it as body fat. In the case of fiber and water, you'd simply use the bathroom more.

As a side note, this is why non-starchy veggies like celery have always been known to help with weight loss. They are basically water and fiber along with a bunch of vitamins and minerals. That entire food group is essentially 100 percent

---

more protein than quinoa. This means you would need to eat 6 servings of quinoa salad to get the same amount of protein you'd get in 1 serving of tuna salad.

inEfficient and therefore helps nourish you with 0 percent chance of causing fat gain.

Moving on to macronutrients, proteins, carbohydrates, and fats: These are broadly defined as compounds that give us energy. But here's the rub: Protein is so inEfficient that I almost wish it wasn't considered a macronutrient. After you eat protein, absolutely no energy is available to your body. Again, *after you eat protein, absolutely no energy is available to your body.* Protein leaves your stomach as amino acids. Amino acids cannot be burned for energy or stored as fat. They are used to repair and create your cells. If protein leaves your stomach as something your body can't use as energy, why is it in the same class as carbohydrates and protein? Because the science of Efficiency is not well known...until now!

I cover the science in detail in my first book, *The Calorie Myth*, so I won't repeat that here, but here's the short version:

- Protein is eaten and enters your stomach.
- Protein is broken down into amino acids. Your body is inEfficient at this. Digestion burns about a third of protein calories.
- Amino acids enter your bloodstream.
- The amino acids then repair and build cells.
- If you have more amino acids than you need, they go to your liver and are converted into glucose. Your body is inEfficient at this. The process burns another third of the protein calories.
- Glucose then enters your bloodstream and can be burned for energy.
- If you have more glucose than you need, it is sent to your fat cells along with insulin and is converted into triglyceride and stored as body fat. Your body is inEfficient at this. The process burns another fourth of the protein calories.

As you can see, it's a long, complex, and calorically costly—that is, inEfficient—road from protein to stored body fat.

As for carbohydrate and fat, both of these macronutrients DO provide energy after leaving your stomach. Your body is pretty Efficient at storing carbohydrate as fat and is very Efficient at storing fat as body fat. Carbohydrates (either sugar or starch) leave your stomach as glucose and are burned for energy or shuttled to fat cells for storage. They do need to be converted into fatty acids before they can be stored, and that is a fairly inEfficient process. However, since that was the only bump on an otherwise short and straight line to your fat cells, let's call sugar and starch Efficient.

Fats leave your stomach as fatty acids and can be burned for energy or stored as body fat. The key here is that there is zero inEfficient processing needed by the body to get fat you eat into your fat cells. It's very Efficient. This does not mean that eating fat makes you fat any more than eating green vegetables makes you green. Remember that the fat you eat could be burned for energy as easily as it is stored. Also keep in mind that fat doesn't trigger the release of the hormone insulin, and that can be very helpful when trying to lower your setpoint. However, it is important to note that processed foods that are *pure* fat—like oils—are easy to overeat and could provide you with way more fatty acids than you need for energy and would then be really Efficiently stored as body fat.

Lots of science here, but just keep doing what you are doing and focus on eating lots of water, fiber, and protein-rich non-starchy vegetables and nutrient-dense protein. Then simply make sure that your fats come in whole-food form so that even they bring water, fiber, and protein along for the ride. An elevated setpoint simply doesn't stand a chance!

Put this all together, and it's clear why eating so much SANE food (Satisfying, unAggressive, Nutritious, and inEfficient) that you are too full for inSANE food heals your metabolism and drives your setpoint down, while starvation dieting harms your metabolism and drives your setpoint up. When you eat as much as you want, whenever you want—as long as it's SANE—your body stops storing fat and burns it instead. You eat more food, maintain a lower setpoint, and slim down naturally.

The next chapters will get into the specifics of the foods that help you do this as simply, quickly, and deliciously as possible.

SANE Points

- *Satiety:* Foods with high Satiety keep you fuller longer and prevent you from eating foods that promote overeating and a high setpoint.
- *Aggression:* Sugars and starches cause your body to release hormones that aggressively store fat and increase your setpoint, while protein, fat, and fiber do not.
- *Nutrition:* The more essential nutrients (vitamins, minerals, essential fatty acids, and essential amino acids) a food provides per calorie, the more it helps to lower your setpoint.
- *Efficiency:* Some things you consume can't be stored as body fat (water and fiber). Some things are hard to store as body fat (protein). Others are easy to store as body fat (sugar, starch, and fat). Focus on water-, fiber-, and protein-rich whole foods and your body will have a hard time storing fat while it lowers your setpoint.

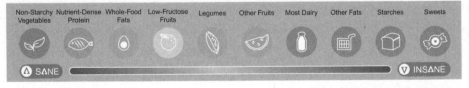

High in water, fiber, and protein   Low in water, fiber, and protein

CHAPTER 4

Non-Starchy Vegetables

From the most militant vegan to the most carnivorous paleo practitioner, the one thing that everyone in the world of nutrition agrees on is that your mother was right: Eat your veggies! In fact, according to a report published in *Food and Chemical Toxicology*, if just half of our population ate 1 extra serving of vegetables every day, 20,000 cases of cancer in this country could be prevented every year (Reiss et al. 2012). Just imagine what magic we could see in our world if we all "go SANE" and conveniently and deliciously devour double-digit servings of veggies daily!

Please don't skip the rest of this chapter. Here's the gist (Warning: It's the furthest thing from sexy but it's the one thing you know will work if you do it): The more veggies you eat, the lower your setpoint will be. Similarly, if you are not happy with your results at any point in time, eat more veggies. If you know anyone who isn't enjoying the body and health they desire, help them eat more veggies.

And we're not talking about just any vegetables. The SANE plan emphasizes "non-starchy vegetables." These are *generally* vegetables that grow aboveground and that you could eat raw. You do not "have to" eat them raw, but you could. For example: spinach, kale, romaine lettuce, broccoli, mushrooms, peppers, zucchini, cucumber, cabbage, and generally vegetables you find in salads.

The best of this bunch are green leafy vegetables. I know that Kermit the Frog thinks that it's not easy being green, but I promise that if you take away nothing else from this book other than eating a lot of green veggies daily, you will lose more weight faster than you ever thought possible, and keep it off forever.

What about other vegetables such as corn, potatoes, and many root vegetables? Applying the "eat raw" standard, these cannot be eaten raw. They are starches, which are extremely easy to overeat because they are dry, relatively low in fiber, and protein poor. When you swap these vegetables out for non-starchy veggies and other water-, fiber-, and protein-rich SANE foods such as seafood, humanely raised meats, low-fructose fruits, nuts, and seeds, your setpoint will be lower and weight loss will be amazing—and lasting.

Non-starchy vegetables are the single most important dietary aspect of this plan—for several reasons.

First, they're loaded with super SANE water, fiber, and, surprisingly, protein.[6] Together, these qualities leave you fuller and less likely to crave starches and sugars—which explains why studies show that people who eat generous portions of a wide variety of vegetables tend to be thinner than people who avoid vegetables.

The specific types of fiber in non-starchy vegetables deserve honorable mention here. Not only do they create a feeling of fullness and stave off hunger pangs, but they also help keep insulin levels in check. In fact, these types of veggies are unAggressive (good), and when you eat them with other foods, they reduce the Aggression of the other foods! The fiber in non-starchy vegetables also helps keep food moving through your digestive tract, while helping to feed the setpoint-lowering form of bacteria in your gut and reducing the inflammation in your brain. Fiber also has the unique ability to bind to and eliminate toxins from the body, including bile acids, which are forerunners to colon tumors and cholesterol formation.

At the risk of stating the obvious, non-starchy vegetables are the most Nutritious (i.e., most nutrients per calorie) foods in the world. Orange vegetables like carrots supply generous amounts of vitamin A, which is important for vision, bone growth, tissue repair, and cellular health, among other benefits. Green vegetables, such as kale and collards, supply iron and calcium, both involved in metabolic health. All vegetables provide health-building phytonutrients.

Also, since they are basically water, fiber, and protein, plus a bunch of setpoint-lowering vitamins and minerals, non-starchy vegetables are essentially impossible for your body to store as fat and are thus the most inEfficient (good) foods in the world. The net effect is that non-starchy vegetables (or "NSV," as we like to call them in the SANE program) optimize and unclog your hormones, reduce inflammation in your brain, and heal your gut. That's why they are your number-one dietary key to lowering your setpoint.

---

[6] Calorie for calorie, spinach contains more protein than many cuts of beef.

SANE NON-STARCHY VEGETABLE CHOICES

The more vegetables you eat, the lower your setpoint and the thinner you'll be. It is impossible to become obese or diabetic if you consistently focus on eating NSVs daily. If after I die, the legacy I leave is that the average daily intake of NSVs increased, I will consider my life a success. Seriously. That's how good they are for you. They can and will save your life while slimming you down.

Back to Kermit: I especially want to emphasize the glory of green vegetables—especially when it comes to diabesity and diabetes. Several years ago, researchers at the University of Leicester reviewed six studies involving more than 220,000 participants. They were searching for a link between eating fruits and vegetables and type 2 diabetes. What they found was that eating more leafy green vegetables, not fruits or any other vegetables, reduced a person's risk of developing type 2 diabetes by 14 percent (Carter et al. 2010). The explanation for the power of vegetables to prevent diabetes has largely to do with the fact that these veggies are packed with the mineral magnesium, which is typically low in people with diabetes. Interestingly, the amount of greens it took to shrink a person's risk for diabetes in this study was just 1½ extra servings a day. That's only as much as one small salad!

For NSVs, the SANE plan categorizes them into "optimal" and "normal." Optimal means that the vegetables in this category have the strongest potential to lower your setpoint. Normal vegetables are other veggies you can eat raw, and, like optimal vegetables, they pack maximum nutrition value with minimal calories, while also helping to lower your SANE setpoint.

Here are some great non-starchy vegetable choices:

Optimal

DEEP GREEN LEAFY VEGETABLES

Deep green vegetables such as those listed below are the best of the best when it comes to NSVs. The reason? Among all vegetables, they are the most Satisfying, the most unAggressive, the most Nutritious, and the most inEfficient. So try to get the bulk of your non-starchy vegetable intake from deep greens. The deeper, the better, too. For example, light green iceberg lettuce isn't as healthy as the deeper green romaine lettuce or the very deep greens such as spinach or kale.

Alfalfa

Arugula

Bok choy

Barley grass*

Brussels sprouts

Chard

Greens (beet, collard, mustard,
    turnip, etc.)

Kale

Kelp

Mixed greens

Moringa*

Neem

Romaine lettuce

Seaweed

Spinach

Spirulina*

Watercress

Wheat grass

These are "supergreens" that also come in powdered supplements, such as whole-food veggie powder. They can be added to smoothies or to water. They are a concentrated source of nutrition and a good way to maximize your veggie and nutrient intake with only a few tablespoons a day.

Normal

VEGGIES YOU CAN EAT RAW

With a few exceptions (such as cauliflower, garlic, and white onions), the richer the color of the NSV, the better it is for you. Choose the colors red, deep yellow, orange, and, of course, dark green. The pigments that make these foods visually appealing contain antioxidants and phytonutrients that help protect against diabetes, cancer, heart disease, and many other health problems.

Alfalfa sprouts

Artichokes

Asparagus

Bean sprouts

Beets

Bell peppers

Broccoli

Cabbage

Carrots

Cauliflower

Celery

Cucumbers

Eggplant

Endive

Garlic

Leeks

Mushrooms

Onions

Peppers (all varieties)

Sugar snap peas

Summer squash (zucchini,
    yellow squash, crookneck,
    pattypan)

Tomatoes

Zucchini

NON-STARCHY VEGETABLE SERVINGS

The next most important issue is: How many servings of non-starchy vegetables should you eat each day?

The answer is at least 10 servings per day. Now let me stop and guess what you're thinking right now. You're thinking there is no way you can eat that many veggies. If we just stopped here, you'd be 100 percent correct because nobody has given you the tools you need to make eating that many veggies practical. However, I promise that this can be easy if you do three things:

1. Cover at least half of your plate with NSVs at each main meal.
2. Read Chapter 7, where you'll learn how to make SANE smoothies, which will give you 6 to 12 servings of optimal NSVs daily. This is easier than you ever thought possible.
3. When eating out—or in—replace starches with NSVs. For example, ask your server to hold the starch and double the veggies, and do this at your dinner table as well.

Be sure to ease your way into eating this many NSVs. Please do not go from no veggies to 12 servings overnight. That will cause all sorts of digestive issues. Add a serving or 2 daily until you reach 12 servings or until you start to have digestive issues. If this happens, add in veggies more gradually, and then when you eat them, eat them more slowly and spaced out over the day.

When thinking about serving sizes, approximations are more than fine. Generally, a serving is about the size of your fist. There are a couple of exceptions: A serving of raw leafy greens is two or three handfuls, and a serving of whole-food veggie powder is only 1 tablespoon. If cooking makes the vegetables shrink (spinach, mushrooms, etc.), then a serving of the cooked NSV is about half the size of your fist.

When we talk about serving sizes, we always frame them in terms of the size of your hand. Why? Because it's ridiculous to think that a serving would be the same size for a giant professional athlete as for a small child. Common sense and science say that serving sizes must be relative to the body they are going into. Because your hand is proportional to your ideal body size, that's how you'll calculate serving sizes.

Again, please free yourself from the stress of precise serving size measures— remember if calorie counting a precise portion control worked, it would have worked already—and focus on eating as many NSVs as possible. Here are some examples of a single serving of NSVs for a 5'4″ woman whose ideal setpoint keeps her at a fit and energetic 140 pounds:

2 to 3 heaping cups of raw leafy
    green vegetables

6 asparagus spears

8 baby carrots

5 large broccoli florets

1 Roma tomato

4 onion slices

5 cherry tomatoes

5 celery sticks

1 whole carrot

1/2 cup cooked spinach

1 tablespoon of whole-food
    veggie powder

FRESH, FROZEN, OR CANNED? ORGANIC?

Both fresh and frozen NSVs are great. Sometimes frozen NSVs can be even better options than their fresh counterparts. This is because frozen vegetables are often flash-frozen in their prime, when their nutrient content is at its peak. If possible, skip canned veggies. They are still better than no veggies, but the way they are typically processed can greatly reduce their Nutrition.

I am often asked if we should eat only organic vegetables. My honest answer? Do whatever works for you and your budget to ensure you get more than 10 servings of NSVs into your body enjoyably every day. If you can afford organic, awesome. If not, fine. The one thing you must not do is eat fewer veggies because of the cost of organic veggies. Ten servings of conventional veggies will always lower your setpoint more than 5 servings of organic veggies. Eat more veggies…whatever it takes!

Raw or Cooked?

Should you cook vegetables or eat them raw? I bet you know what I'm going to say here. Your top priority is eating at least 10 servings of NSVs a day, so do whatever is necessary within reason to get 10-plus servings into your body. In an ideal world, you would not only eat a variety of NSVs, but you would also eat them in a variety of ways: raw, steamed, boiled, sautéed, roasted, and so forth. The only cooking methods to avoid are frying and overcooking. Among other issues, the excessive heating from both destroys much of what makes veggies so very SANE.

DON'T I NEED TO SAVE SOME ROOM FOR STARCH?

The scientifically unquestionable answer is no.

I am going to let you in on a little secret: Carbohydrates—which includes starches (along with sugars)—are not essential. There are essential fats. There are essential amino acids (proteins). There are essential vitamins and minerals. But there is no such thing as an essential carbohydrate. Remember that during digestion, carbohydrates are converted into glucose. If you never ate any carbs, your body would simply create glucose from other nutrients you eat, such as protein.

Even our own carbohydrate-loving USDA noted it in its *Dietary Reference Intakes for Energy, Carbohydrate, Fiber, Fat, Fatty Acids, Cholesterol, Protein, and Amino Acids*: "The lower limit of dietary carbohydrate compatible with life apparently is zero, provided that adequate amounts of protein and fat are consumed."

I am not sure why they stuck the word *apparently* in there, but oh well. The point is that there is no biological reason to eat carbohydrates unless they help you to consume *required* vitamins, minerals, fat, or protein. Guess which forms of carbohydrates do that better than any other? Non-starchy vegetables.

Also, free your mind from the simple carbohydrates versus complex carbohydrate complexity. This distinction causes confusion. For example, SANE low-fructose fruits contain simple carbohydrates, while inSANE starches contain complex carbohydrates. Oh no! Not so fast. The complex carbohydrates in rice, cereal, crackers, potatoes, and wheat bread are all *more* hormonally harmful (they all raise our blood sugar more) than the simple carbohydrates found in low-fructose fruits. You can avoid all this confusion by forgetting about simple vs. complex carbs completely and focusing instead on enjoying more water-, fiber-, and protein-rich SANE foods.

Finally, let's cover "low-carb" real quick. There's nothing wrong with low-carb diets, and this isn't a low-carb diet. SANE eating is an optimal carb diet. You are eating A LOT of the forms of carbs that are most effective at lowering your setpoint. This generally amounts to between 70 and 125 grams daily of the most therapeutic carbs in the world. Low-carb or ketogenic diets specify under 50 grams of carbs daily. Just like you could be SANE paleo, SANE kosher, or SANE vegetarian, you could be SANE low-carb/ketogenic, but SANE "out of the box" isn't low-carb/ketogenic.

Your goal here isn't to adhere to any diet dogma. Your goal is to lower your setpoint using the foods proven to do that. As you'll see, the tremendous flexibility around which of those foods you choose make SANE living compatible with just about any other dietary lifestyle. However, one thing is nonnegotiable when it comes to your health, happiness, and lowered setpoint. By now I bet you know what it is: lots of non-starchy veggies!!

SANE Points

- Cover half of your plate with NSVs.
- Drink yummy veggie-packed SANE smoothies.
- If a non-starchy can't be eaten raw, it is probably not SANE.
- Stick with fresh or frozen, conventional or organic.
- Greens are great. The deeper the color, the higher the SANEity.
- A serving is about one to three handfuls, with certain exceptions.
- Work your way toward eating 10-plus servings a day of non-starchy vegetables. The more servings of these foods you eat daily, the lower your setpoint and the slimmer and healthier you will be for life.

CHAPTER 5

Nutrient-Dense Proteins

The second most important nutritional strategy for lowering your setpoint is to enjoy 3 to 6 servings of nutrient-dense proteins, along with your non-starchy vegetables. Protein, from the Greek word meaning "of prime importance," is...wait for it...of prime importance. One of the main reasons for its Rockstar Satiety status is that protein makes you feel fuller faster and longer than any other source of calories. The more protein you eat (to a point), the harder it will be to overeat.

Nutrient-dense protein is also excellently unAggressive. Unlike starches and sugars, it does not flood your bloodstream with glucose and therefore doesn't spike levels of the hormone insulin. In fact, it promotes the production of the "antidote" to insulin—the hormone glucagon, which helps *unlock* fat stores.

Nutrient-dense protein is also an excellent source of some of the most biologically potent nutrients, including certain essential amino acids, essential fatty acids, B vitamins, and minerals such as zinc and iron.

Plus, it has a tremendously beneficial impact on hormonal health, especially when it comes to optimizing your balance of the sex hormones estrogen and testosterone. According to researcher James O'Keefe, MD, at the Mid America Heart Institute, eating a good amount of protein at regular intervals can not only help you feel satisfied, but also increase your metabolic rate, improve your cholesterol ratio and your insulin sensitivity, and help speed weight loss.

Finally, you'll recall that protein is very inEfficient. If you exchange calories from carbs or fat for calories from protein, you will lose weight even though your calorie count is unchanged. Why? Even though you are eating the same number of calories, a larger portion of those calories are super inEfficient at becoming body fat (yea, protein!), and you drop weight.

Nutrient-dense proteins have a profound effect on lowering your setpoint. To make the most of this effect, let's cover how to select nutrient-dense proteins. Just like a calorie isn't a calorie, protein isn't protein; quality varies wildly. Here's how to make the SANEest high-quality, most setpoint-lowering protein picks.

SANE NUTRIENT-DENSE PROTEIN CHOICES

Odds are, you've heard protein described in terms such as "complete" or "incomplete," which refer to a protein's amino acid profile. Animal sources of protein are more "complete" than plant sources of protein. There's also a little-known measure of how much of a given source of protein your body can use. It's called *biological availability*. Higher is better. Animal sources of protein have a higher *biological availability* than plant sources of protein. Put these both together and you see why you may have rightly been told that animal sources of protein are "better" than plant sources. From an "is the protein able to repair and build cells" perspective, this is unequivocally true. From an animal rights perspective or environmental perspective, well, that's a whole different book, so let's stay focused on your best nutrient-dense protein picks to specifically lower your setpoint.

To select the most effective proteins to lower your setpoint, you must be able to identify your favorite "concentrated proteins" and "nutrient-dense proteins." Concentrated sources of protein are foods that have more calories coming from protein than from fat or carbohydrates, and whose protein can be readily used by the body (i.e., complete and high biological availability). Here are some examples of highly concentrated sources of SANE protein:

Seafood: 51 to 94 percent protein

Egg whites: 91 percent protein

White meat with or without skin: 51 to 80 percent protein

Dark meat without skin: 60 percent protein

Nonfat cottage cheese: 60 to 85 percent protein

Nonfat plain Greek yogurt: 60 to 70 percent protein

Lean (ideally grass-fed) red meat: 51 to 75 percent protein

Low-sugar casein or whey protein powder: 70 percent or more protein

Plant proteins are fine, but they just aren't highly concentrated sources of protein. Also, sources of protein that contain good amounts of fats or carbs are not deal breakers and can be fine, too, but they just aren't *highly concentrated* sources of protein. For example, consider eggs. Because 63 percent of the calories in an egg comes from fat while only 35 percent comes from protein, eggs are not a concentrated source of protein. Eggs are still SANE. But including the yolks tips eggs over into whole-food fat territory, whereas egg whites are legitimately considered concentrated protein because they are more than 90 percent protein.

Here are some examples of fairly concentrated sources of SANE proteins:[7]

- Dark-meat poultry with skin: 45 percent protein
- Moderately fatty (ideally grass-fed) red meat: 40 to 60 percent protein
- Eggs: 35 percent protein
- Low-sugar vegetarian protein powders (rice, pea, or hemp): 50 percent or more protein

Everything else is not even close to being a concentrated source of protein. An example would be common dairy products such as milk. They contain mostly fat and sugar. Beans are mostly carbohydrate. Nuts are more than 70 percent fat. Again, being mostly fat or carbohydrate does not necessarily make these foods bad; it just makes it inaccurate to call them concentrated sources of protein.

Let's next define "nutrient dense." These are proteins with as much protein, vitamins, and minerals *per calorie* as possible. If you have two instances of a food that are the same in every way except that one contains more fat than the other (e.g., fat-free versus full-fat cottage cheese), divide the protein, vitamins, and minerals in a serving by the calories in a serving and the option with less fat is the more nutrient-dense source of protein. This is not to say that the full-fat versions of these foods should be avoided; rather, if your goal is to pick a food that maximizes protein, vitamin, and mineral intake, you should pick leaner options. Concentrated sources of protein also happen to be nutrient-dense proteins.

---

[7] Soy is never recommended if your goal is to lower your setpoint. It has counterproductive effects on your hormones and the very limited amount of protein it provides is of low quality.

When considering protein options, keep in mind that just because a food has some protein in it does not qualify it as a setpoint-lowering source of protein. Next time you are at the grocery store and you see an advertisement saying "high in protein," you can double-check that with these quick tips:

- If grams of carbs are greater than grams of protein, it's not a nutrient-dense protein.
- If you divide grams of protein by 2 and that number is less than the grams of fat, it's not a nutrient-dense protein.

Also, not all proteins are created equal—back to complete versus incomplete and biological availability—and many of the "good sources of protein" you hear of are about as good at meeting your protein needs as ketchup is good at meeting your non-starchy vegetable needs.

OPTIMAL NUTRIENT-DENSE PROTEIN CHOICES

Optimal nutrient-dense proteins are like the Navy Seals of the protein world. They do everything good that protein does but better than all other sources of protein. They are the most concentrated and nutrient dense of all proteins. This does not mean "normal" nutrient-dense proteins are bad. Normal nutrient-dense proteins are setpoint-lowering superstars. We're talking about going from an A to an A+ with these optimal choices. Also, "humanely raised" proteins are recommended. They tend to be leaner, higher in nutrition, and free of hormones and other additives. Plus, destroying the environment and animal cruelty are both insane and inSANE.

Here are your best choices:

Optimal Nutrient-Dense Proteins

(Shellfish, fatty fish, and organ meats)

Anchovies	Salmon
Clams	Sardines
Liver	Sea bass
Mussels	Tuna
Oysters	

A flood of research suggests that in addition to all the protein-related benefits discussed above, consuming seafood frequently can drop your risk of the vast majority of diseases plaguing us today. Do your best to eat seafood daily. Not a few times per week. Daily. This is simple because cooking seafood is a snap. Place some fish and some seasoning in a pan or baking dish and heat it. You will be delighted when you eat it. Canned seafood options such as canned salmon, tuna, and sardines require no cooking and provide inexpensive portable protein. The recipe section is filled with delicious ways to cook seafood and other SANE proteins.

Normal Nutrient-Dense Proteins*

(Humanely raised seafood and meats)

Bison

Catfish

Chicken

Cod

Cornish hen

Cottage cheese, nonfat

Crab

Croaker

Egg whites + whole eggs

Elk

Flounder

Grass-fed beef

Haddock

Halibut

Ham

Herring

Lamb

Lean conventional beef

Lobster

Mackerel

Mahi-mahi

Octopus

Organ meats

Plain Greek yogurt, nonfat

Pollock

Pork

Protein powders (unflavored):
   clean hemp, pea, rice, and
   whey protein powders

Rabbit

Scallops

Shad

Shrimp

Snapper

Sole

Squid (calamari)

Swordfish

Tilapia

Tofu

Trout

Turkey

Venison

Whitefish

The Mercury Issue

Seafood is super SANE. Mercury is not. That's why your SANEst seafood choices should be low in mercury. Generally speaking, avoid these higher mercury options: shark, swordfish, king mackerel, and tilefish.

But much more importantly, please do not throw the baby out with the bathwater when it comes to seafood. If you have any mercury-related concerns with eating SANE seafood daily, please ask yourself two questions: How many people do you know whose lives have been severely negatively impacted by mercury? and How many people do you know whose lives have been severely negatively impacted by overweight or diabetes?

For the vast majority of people, the benefits of eating SANE seafood vastly outweigh anything related to mercury. In fact, most credible health organizations point to the overwhelming evidence that increasing the amount of seafood we eat—along with more veggies—is one of the most important things we can do to improve health and lose weight.

In sum: Allowing mercury mythology to distract you from the metabolic miracle you'll enjoy with SANE seafood is a bit like worrying about bird poop on your car's windshield while the engine is on fire. Please don't allow something minor to distract you from addressing something major.

NUTRIENT-DENSE PROTEIN SERVING SIZES

Each day, eat 3 to 6 servings of nutrient-dense protein—which is as easy as filling a third of your plate with nutrient-dense proteins at breakfast, lunch, and dinner.

This ensures that you get 30 to 55 grams of protein at each meal, or a per day tally of between 100 grams and 200 grams of protein, depending on your size and activity level. A five-foot 110-pound sedentary woman would be fine with about 100 grams, while a six-foot 195-pound man who exercises smarter (the SANE approach to exercise you'll learn about in Part 4) should take in about 200 grams.

If you eat less than about 30 grams of protein in a sitting, you won't enjoy all the benefits protein has to offer. That's because when you eat about 30 grams (or more) of protein, the concentration of a specific amino acid in your blood, called leucine, becomes high enough to cause your body to refresh and renew your lean tissue. The technical term for this is *muscle protein synthesis*—your body is rebuilding itself, and without activating this mechanism at least three times a day, you are missing out on all sorts of metabolic benefits and risk losing about 5 percent of your muscle tissue per decade. This condition is known as *sarcopenia*. It can be thought of as osteoporosis for muscles, but you'll avoid it easily thanks to your SANE approach to protein.

If you think that's promising, just wait till you see how protein literally causes you to burn more by eating more. Researchers at the University of Illinois have found that when you eat a SANE quantity and quality of protein daily, you can trigger your body to replace about 250 grams of old tissue with robust new tissue each day (Layman n.d.). This process can cause you to burn up to 700 more calories daily. It is so calorically costly, that it causes your cells to generate more mitochondria (metabolic power plants)—a reaction once thought possible only via intense exercise. This literally means that by eating more protein you can cause your body to burn more calories than you'd burn by jogging for 2 hours!

If you follow the serving guides and recipes on the plan, and enjoy nutrient-dense protein at each main meal, you'll consume just the right amount of protein and be surprised at how full you are and how much better you feel and look long-term—all while your setpoint plummets and your body burns radically more calories automatically.

In general, a serving size is a little larger than your palm. Here are some additional examples of serving sizes:

- A piece of humanely raised meat, poultry, or fish about the size of your hand
- A heaping cup of nonfat cottage cheese or plain nonfat Greek yogurt
- 1 whole egg + 5 egg whites
- 8 egg whites
- 1 can of tuna
- 4 tablespoons of protein powder

Facts and Fiction about Protein

Let's sort through the fact and fiction about protein, tackling the four most common misconceptions and setting the record straight on this essential setpoint-lowering food.

Fiction: Too much protein harms the kidneys and heart.

Fact: This myth is not borne out in randomized controlled testing, say experts from Harvard to Finland. Hundreds of studies show positive health benefits and body-fat loss stemming from the level of protein intake we're discussing.

A report from Colorado State University, for example, cites a large body of experimental evidence that demonstrates a higher intake of lean animal protein reduces the risk for cardiovascular disease, hypertension, dyslipidemia, obesity, insulin resistance, and osteoporosis while not impairing kidney function (Cordain and Campbell n.d.).

So how did the fiction that protein is bad get started? I believe that it arose from studies in which animals were fed extreme amounts of low-quality sources of protein and then experienced problems. But rather than proving protein is harmful, these studies led to the discovery that until an inactive person exceeds 2 grams of protein per pound of body weight per day, we only get healthier and slimmer by enjoying additional nutrient-dense proteins.

Luckily, it is impossible to consistently eat too much nutrient-dense protein. Your stomach would explode. Worrying about eating too much whole-food nutrient-dense protein is a bit like worrying about drinking too much water. Can it be done? Yes. Will you do it? No.

Fiction: Meat is unhealthy.

Fact: While some might argue against eating meat for environmental or ethical reasons, science proves there is nothing inherently unhealthy about humanely raised *nutrient-dense* meat. In fact, low levels of animal protein have been associated with an *increased* risk of strokes.

Academic work that cautions against meat is referring to the inSANE heavily processed meat such as hot dogs, bologna, pink slime, and so on—diets in which people replace vitamin- and mineral-rich foods with non-nutrient-dense meat.

These works are quite right—you should not do that. You should eat the most nutrient-dense food possible—and that includes many forms of seafood and meat. If you have any doubts, consider the *Journal of the American Medical Association*'s review of 147 diet and health studies (Willett and Hu 2002). That review found zero correlation between meat consumption and heart disease. Nutrient-dense meat is not unhealthy!

Fiction: Protein causes cancer.

Fact: This one hits home for me and needs to be put to bed once and for all. It is a misunderstanding that comes up because high-quality protein promotes the repair and growth of cells—all cells. Therefore, if a person *already has cancer*, excessive protein can cause those cells to grow along with every other cell in the body. Does that mean protein caused the cancer? No. As University of Illinois nutrition researcher Chris Masterjohn, PhD, notes in his review of the research related to protein and cancer, "low-protein diets depressed normal growth, increased the susceptibility to many toxins, killed toxin-exposed animals earlier, induced fatty liver, and increased the development of pre-cancerous lesions" (Masterjohn 2010).

The bottom line is that eating protein causes cancer the way watering gardens causes weeds. Just as you don't effectively avoid weeds by depriving your garden of water, you don't effectively avoid cancer by depriving your body of protein. You're better served cultivating a metabolic system robust enough to ward off intruders in the first place. Fortunately, that's exactly what water-, fiber-, and protein-rich SANE foods do.

Fiction: Protein promotes osteoporosis.

Fact: This misinformation may spring from the fact that digesting protein requires more calcium than the digestion of fat or carbohydrates. Certain individuals claim this finding shows that eating a lot of protein will suck calcium from your bones—but in the case of the SANE lifestyle, these concerns are not valid.

First, you are not eating "a lot" of protein. Second, because you are eating so many non-starchy vegetables, your body has no need to take calcium from your bones, since your non-starchy vegetable intake provides at least 150 percent more calcium than the typical U.S. diet. (For example, leafy green vegetables are excellent sources of calcium. Calorie for calorie, spinach provides nearly twice as much calcium as reduced-fat milk.) Third, protein digestion does not negatively affect bones if intake of the mineral phosphorus is increased, and the SANE eating plan does that. Finally, while more protein increases the need for calcium, it also increases your ability to absorb calcium. When more protein is taken in, the body automatically makes better use of calcium.

CAN I BE A SANE VEGAN OR VEGETARIAN?

Absolutely! Vegetarians and vegans can enjoy a Satisfying, unAggressive, Nutritious, and inEfficient lifestyle as much as anyone else. Replacing starches and sweets with non-starchy vegetables, nutrient-dense non-animal protein, whole-food fats, and low-fructose fruits is as healthy and slimming for those who eat animal products as it is for those who abstain.

If you are a vegetarian, you can skip the rest of this section because, generally speaking, seafood is the best source of nutrient-dense protein on the planet.

Admittedly, there is a wrinkle for vegans because not all proteins are created equally. One of the major reasons we need to eat protein is that the body requires certain amino acids. Not all proteins are the same when it comes to the quality and quantity of essential amino acids they provide (complete versus incomplete), or if the body can use the amino acids provided (biological availability). Plant sources of protein are poor at both of these when compared to animal sources of protein.

That said, vegans read on because I have much respect for you (it takes a very disciplined person to never eat any animal foods), and it is definitely possible to consume a SANE quantity and quality of protein from only plants. Protein powders made from rice, pea, or hemp protein are good substitutions. Also, mollusks such as oysters, clams, and mussels are the most optimal sources of nutrient-dense protein, so if the absence of a central nervous system makes these living beings closer to plants than to animals, you will be healthier and slimmer if you are able to add them to your diet. I also advise vegetarians to take a branched-chain amino acid supplement to address the suboptimal amino acid profile of plants.

Please always remember that a SANE lifestyle *is* plant-based. In fact, if you are a SANE omnivore, you will eat more plants than an inSANE herbivore. Your giant plates will be overflowing with mostly non-starchy vegetables, and a large chunk of our calories will come from plant fats such as cocoa, coconut, avocado, flax, and chia. As Joel Fuhrman, MD, states elegantly in his article "What You Need to Know about Vegetarian or Vegan Diets" on his website: "You can achieve the benefits of a vegetarian diet, without being a vegetarian or a vegan."

Nutrient-dense protein is delicious, satisfying, and second only to non-starchy vegetables when it comes to lowering your setpoint and living radically better. If you eat about 30 grams of nutrient-dense protein and at least 3 servings of NSVs every time you eat, it is impossible *not* to be slim and healthy. Period. If you find someone who says they consistently do those two things and isn't at their ideal weight, please let me know at FibAlert@SANESolution.com.

SANE Points

- Nutrient-dense protein is super SANE and essential to lowering your setpoint. It keeps you full, heals your hormones, provides abundant essential nutrition, and is hard to store as fat.
- Eat protein in 30- to 55-gram servings evenly throughout the day, for a total of 100 to 200 grams of protein per day. Nutrient-dense protein should cover a third of your plate.
- Enjoy seafood daily (ideally sources higher in omega-3s and lower in mercury, such as salmon, sardines, anchovies, oysters, etc.).
- High-quality, nutrient-dense sources of protein are critical. If you avoid animal products, you can still be SANE.

CHAPTER 6

Whole-Food Fats and Sweets

One of the best things about SANE eating is that you can enjoy every taste (sweet, sour, salty, bitter, and savory/fatty) in abundance while lowering your setpoint. In your Setpoint Diet you will enjoy setpoint-lowering sources of all the flavors while eliminating any food cravings and addictions.

Let's start with your SANE approach to burning fat with fat thanks to your discovery of whole-food fats.

SANE WHOLE-FOOD FATS

These are foods found directly in nature that contain more calories from fat than from protein or carbohydrate. Nuts, seeds, eggs, olives, and avocados are good examples. Oils are not. If you're trying to figure out whether a food that gets most of its calories from fat is a "whole-food" fat, just ask yourself: Can you find it directly in nature? Nuts, yes. Olives, yes. Vegetable oil, no. Olive oil, no (gasp!).

The Setpoint Diet puts a premium on whole-food fats because they contain everything that's nutritious about the oil—and more. Far too much attention is paid to oils, while the whole foods they are found in are ignored despite being unequivocally better for you. Oils are previously whole foods with all the water, fiber, and protein processed out. Why is the media praising processed forms of fat with all things SANE stripped from them instead of heaping accolades on their far more therapeutic whole-food origins?

One of the neatest things about getting most of your calories from whole-food fats instead of starch and sugar is that this alone fundamentally changes the way your metabolism works, transforming your body from being good at storing fat to being good at burning fat. When you eat these whole foods in place of starches and sweets, your body starts to prefer burning fat for fuel instead of sugar. As you go SANE and get smarter about physical activity, you begin to burn more calories than you take in—but you won't feel hungry and your body isn't slowing down. Why? Because it's full of nutrients and still has plenty of its preferred fuel. Sure, the fuel is body fat sitting on your hips instead of bread that just passed through your lips, but why would your body care? It has enough nutrition and enough energy on hand to keep you at your best.

Just the opposite happens if you regularly eat starches and sweets. Calories from sugar and starches slow your metabolism and shift the body into a fat-storage mode, resulting in increased hunger and cravings.

If you burn more calories than you're eating, your body looks around for its preferred fuel source—sugar (remember, starch means lots of sugars mashed together)—but doesn't find any. This deficit makes it demand more sugar and you experience this as crazy carb cravings. Even if you're able to fight through these all-encompassing cravings and hunger pangs, you know what happens next: Your body burns fewer calories.

But what if there's still a sugar shortage? Your body turns toward burning vital muscle tissue.

Eventually, it will get to burning body fat—but why not skip the whole "feel hungry and terrible while your body cannibalizes your muscles" part? Far from *making* you heavier, eating whole-food fats instead of starches and sweets enables you to healthfully *burn* body fat.

I know that it can be hard to let go of the theory that fat is bad for your waistline and for your health. Good news: *Modern science* (versus outdated myths) proves that it is not bad for you. Whole foods—which are generally SANE foods—contain fat. Whole foods were the only thing our ancestors ate for 99.8 percent of our history. How could the only foods available to us for 99.8 percent of our history harm you? If anything, you will thrive on foods that contain fats.

Then there is the crazier theory that fat is fattening. This has never been scientifically demonstrated, despite more than a billion dollars' worth of research attempting to prove it. Indeed, researchers have proved that some types of fat help burn body fat and boost health.

Almonds—a SANE whole-food fat—are a good example. In a randomized study of 48 volunteers with elevated LDL cholesterol, Pennsylvania State University researchers demonstrated that eating 1.5 ounces of almonds daily burned belly fat, plus reduced artery-clogging cholesterol over a 6-week period (Berryman et al. 2015).

Diets high in fat don't make you heavier. In fact, among European women, the data show that the more dietary fat women eat, the less body fat they carry. And any attempts to limit supposedly dangerous saturated fats by increasing carbohydrates just make health matters way worse—increasing triglycerides and decreasing healthy HDL cholesterol, raising glycemic load and insulin levels, and increasing the risk of diabetes, diabesity, and heart disease. Harvard researchers stress that the greatest hope related to fats in the diet points not to decreasing them but to *increasing* them: "Studies and…trials have provided strong evidence that a higher intake of [omega-3] fatty acids from fish or plant sources lowers risk of coronary heart disease" (Hu et al. 2001).

Finally, because of our fear of fat, there has been a decline in the proportion of fat in our diet, partly because food manufacturers rushed to create "low-fat" foods, which were really loaded with carbs specifically engineered to use taste to make up for the lack of fat. Tellingly, this dietary blunder has been accompanied by the largest spike in obesity and disease rates in history. Research from Harvard Medical School blames the decades-long emphasis on dietary fat reduction for having distracted us in the fight against the true causes of obesity (Ludwig 2016).

As you begin to eat whole-food fats, you'll start limiting your consumption of "processed fats." These include vegetable oils, butter, margarine, mayonnaise, bottled salad dressings, sour cream, and so forth. Again, all these fats, particularly oils, are processed derivatives of whole foods. They contain no water, no fiber, and no protein and are therefore not substances you need to eat. They just aren't SANE.

Take soybean oil, for example, whose consumption has skyrocketed about 116,300 percent over the past century. It is not a whole food and is actually a highly refined product of soy—which can block the synthesis of thyroid hormones and interfere with metabolism, both of which can elevate your setpoint.

Are you thinking: But what about olive oil and coconut oil? Aren't we told they're good for us? Yes, but that's relative to other oils. Think about this in the same way you think about whole grains. Whole grains are better than refined grains, but that doesn't mean they are *good* for you. Same thing with oil: Olive oil and coconut oil are much better for you than other oils (soybean, corn, vegetable, and so on), but whole olives and whole coconuts are dramatically better for you than any oil. Why? Thanks to their higher water, fiber, and protein content, whole olives and whole coconuts are more Satiating (good), less Aggressive (good), more Nutritious (good), and less Efficient (good) than the oil extracted from them.

If you really want to throw a wrench into what the Internet says about "healthy oils," it's interesting to compare them to sugar. Specifically, how is sugar produced? Take a whole food that contains sugar—say, sugarcane—and then process it until all that's left is refined sugar. How are even "healthy oils" produced? Take a whole food that contains oil—olives, for example—and then process it until all that's left is refined oil. Does this mean oils are as bad for you as sugar? No. Does it mean that you can lower your setpoint faster if you get your fats from whole foods instead of oils? Yes.

Stable natural oils such as coconut oil and olive oil are fine when used sparingly for cooking, but whole-food fats are best for eating. Need a little oil to make your non-starchy vegetables delicious? All good. Simply keep in mind that anyone telling you to eat a tablespoon of coconut oil per day rather than eating more coconut meat may be more interested in selling you coconut oil than in your health!

YOUR SANE WHOLE-FOOD FAT CHOICES

Although there are many healthy sources of whole-food fats, some are especially beneficial. Rising to the top are cocoa/cacao, coconut, chia seeds, flax seeds, eggs, avocados, and olives.

Cocoa/cacao and coconut are wonderful ways to indulge your cravings for sweets. Beyond their deliciousness, these foods are health and fat-loss powerhouses. Natural and undutched cocoa/cacao is one of the richest sources of antioxidants, polyphenols, and flavanols (hard-to-come-by healthy things) in the world. By contrast, dutched or dutch-processed cocoa/cacao has been treated with chemicals and has lost much of its health benefit. Cocoa is also packed with filling fiber and essential vitamins and nutrients.

Coconut is home for a rare therapeutic type of fat: medium-chain tri-glycerides (MCTs), which have been shown to boost metabolism. MCTs are burned up rather quickly in the body for energy. And coconuts have fairly strong antiviral properties.

Flax seeds and chia seeds are rich sources of fiber, vitamins, and minerals, and are useful sources of omega-3 fats, extremely beneficial fats that have been shown to benefit almost every aspect of human cardiac, metabolic, and neurological health. Keep in mind that flax seeds need to be milled into a flourlike powder in order for your body to be able to use their abundant nutrition.

Also, while I love chia and flax, remember that the omega-3 fats found in plants (alpha-linolenic acid [ALA]) are 5 to 10 times less helpful than omega-3 fats found in animals (eicosapentaenoic acid [EPA] and docosahexaenoic acid [DHA]). Yet another reason to enjoy seafood every day whenever possible. In fact, animal-based omega-3s are literally therapeutic...that is, you can actually get a prescription for them!

Now let's talk about eggs. Holy moly. If there was an award for most confusing food, eggs would get it...until now. Here's why: Eggs are high in cholesterol. This *had been* the source of all the confusion. Fortunately, the research community has recently achieved cholesterol clarity. Eating SANE amounts of cholesterol is in no way, shape, or form bad for you. Thanks to that scientific fact, eggs become simple. They are a superfood. Think about it like this: One egg contains everything needed to create a life. What other food can we say that about? Eggs stand alone and are super SANE whole-food fats.

Then there are delightful whole-food fats like avocado and olives rich in setpoint-lowering monounsaturated fats. A 2013 study, published in the *Critical Reviews in Food Science and Nutrition*, reported that avocado eaters are slimmer, with thinner waistlines, and have normal levels of cholesterol. Olives contain healthy fat that helps to lower LDL or bad cholesterol and increase HDL or good cholesterol in your blood (Dreher and Davenport 2013). Remember, everything that makes olive oil "good" *and so much more* is found in whole olives.

Just like with non-starchy vegetables and nutrient-dense protein, you can pick your favorite whole-food fats from "optimal" and "normal" categories. Optimal simply means that the food supplies the maximum amount of nutrition per calorie; normal is still SANE but yields slightly less nutrition per calories.

Optimal

(Uniquely Nutritious superfoods)

Avocados

Chia seeds

Cocoa/cacao

Cocoa/cacao nibs

Coconut

Coconut flour

Coconut milk

Eggs

Flax seeds

Macadamia nuts

Olives

Normal

(Most raw nuts and seeds)

Almonds

Brazil nuts

Cashews

Chestnuts

Hazelnuts

Hemp seeds

Kola nuts

Pecans

Pistachios

Pumpkin seeds

Sesame seeds

Squash seeds

Sunflower seeds

Walnuts

Whole-Food Fats from Nutrient-Dense Protein

You'll also be enjoying whole-food fats from SANE proteins, namely salmon, halibut, sardines, mackerel, and other fish—all loaded with the previously mentioned therapeutic EPA and DHA forms of omega-3 fats. These build brain-cell membranes, reduce neuroinflammation, and promote new brain-cell formation. They also help regulate hormones and lower your setpoint. In a 2015 study in *Molecular Nutrition and Food Research*, omega-3s latched onto receptors on fat cells and prevented weight gain and inflammation (Smith et al. 2015). Fish oil and other healthy fats also improve insulin sensitivity and adiponectin levels. Personally, if I could recommend only one supplement, it without question would be a tablespoon of EPA- and DHA-rich fish oil daily.

WHOLE-FOOD FATS SERVING SIZES

For better setpoint lowering and maximal health, eat 1 to 6 servings a day of whole-food fats. A serving of plant fats such as nuts and seeds is generally a small handful or 3 tablespoons. If the nuts are mashed into butter (natural almond butter), a serving is the size of a Ping-Pong ball, or 2 tablespoons. When combined with NSVs and nutrient-dense protein, a serving of a whole-food fat is filling. Most people will stop eating naturally at 2 servings in a single sitting, anyway.

Here are other examples of serving sizes:

½ cup of coconut flour	¼ cup chocolate bites or cacao
¼ cup shredded unsweetened	nibs
coconut	¼ cup flax seeds
2 cups SANE coconut milk	½ avocado
¼ cup chia seeds	

Note: You can eat "unlimited" olives and cocoa. They're so nutritionally dense and satisfying that you can consider them a "free food."

SANE LOW-FRUCTOSE FRUITS

I'll go out on a limb and say that 99.99 percent of people have been told setpoint-elevating misinformation about fruit. This is all caused by "experts" being sloppy with language. They tell us "eat more fruits and veggies." They treat fruits and veggies as one food group. At the risk of stating the obvious: Fruits are not veggies.

For example, grapes contain 24 times more sugar per calorie than kale. If you get "five a day," as the common adage recommends, from the *fruit* grapes, you will become diabetic as you bathe yourself in the same amount of sugar found in three full-sized cans of Coke! If you get "five a day" from the vegetable kale, you will take in essentially no sugar. Fruits and veggies are not the same, and your body and health will never be the same now that you know that.

Does this mean all fruits are off-limits? No. It does mean that if you think about fruits as "vegetables with WAY more sugar," your setpoint will thank you. Now, as with every other type of food, not all fruits are created equal. Some fruits, such as acai berries and goji berries, are much lower in sugar and much higher in setpoint-lowering substances than other fruits.

A little higher in sugar, but still SANE are common berries, citrus fruits, and certain melons. However, fruits such as bananas, pineapples, grapes, and watermelon are best thought of as nature's candy. They are not SANE.

But wait! Don't all fruits contain vitamins? Yes. However, if you add a vitamin pill to a glass of sugary soda, did you make the soda good for you? No. And the similarities to soda don't stop there. Ever heard of high-fructose corn syrup (HFCS)? It's the primary sweetener in soda. Guess what the primary source of sugar in fruit is: fructose. Guess what form of sugar is particularly damaging to your setpoint: fructose.

Glucose and fructose act much differently in your body. While glucose passes directly through the liver and is used by any cell in the body, fructose can stick around in your liver and get converted quickly into triglycerides—a fat in the blood that's made when you consume excess sugar (including fructose). High levels of triglycerides are associated with abdominal obesity, diabetes, insulin resistance, low levels of high-density lipoproteins (the "good" cholesterol), and a higher risk of heart disease.

Fructose has been found to have a strong fat-storing effect on the body. Research conducted at the University of Texas Southwestern Medical Center and published in 2008 demonstrated the surprising speed at which human bodies turn fructose into body fat. For the study, researchers fed six healthy volunteers three different breakfast drinks—one containing 100 percent glucose, one containing 50 percent glucose and 50 percent fructose, and the third containing 25 percent glucose and 75 percent fructose. They also ate a carefully controlled lunch over several weeks.

The researchers then measured the conversion of the sugars to fat in the liver. They also looked at how the morning drink influenced the metabolism of foods eaten later in the day. What they found was intriguing: "Lipogenesis"—the conversion of sugars into body fat—increased significantly when the breakfast drinks contained mostly fructose. Also, when fructose was eaten with fat or before fat was consumed, the fat was more likely to be stored rather than burned.

Those fruit carbs (fructose) entered the body as sugars; the liver took the molecules apart, and put them back together to build fats. All this happened within 4 hours after the fructose drink. As a result, when the next meal was eaten, fat eaten at lunch was more likely to be stored than burned (Parks et al. 2008). Fructose is very Efficient at becoming body fat, and worse, it makes everything else you eat more Efficient at becoming body fat, too!

Also, HFCS can trigger leptin resistance, as reported by a study in the *American Journal of Physiology* (Shapiro et al. 2008). It also contributes to insulin resistance and neuroinflammation. Your hunger signals can get mixed up as a result. You may overeat the wrong foods and ultimately elevate your setpoint.

The bottom line is that to lower your setpoint, lose all the weight you've ever wanted to, and keep the body from storing fat, enjoy low-fructose fruits instead of high-fructose fruits.

SANE LOW-FRUCTOSE FRUIT CHOICES

Same optimal versus normal deal here. Optimal are fruits that contain the least fructose and the most nutrition. Normal are SANE, just not as SANE as the optimal choices.

Optimal*

(Least sugar, most nutrition)

Acai berries	Noni fruit
Goji berries	Purple aronia
Mangosteen	Lemons

You may recognize these fruits as "superfruits," and they are—singled out for packing a bigger nutritional punch because they contain high levels of vitamins, fiber, and antioxidants that are thought to help protect against cancer and heart disease.

Normal

(Berries, citrus, and others)

Apricots	Guava
Blackberries	Honeydew melon
Blueberries	Limes
Boysenberries	Nectarines
Cantaloupe	Papayas
Casaba melons	Peaches
Cherries	Raspberries
Cranberries	Strawberries
Grapefruit	

SANE LOW-FRUCTOSE FRUIT SERVING SIZES

If you enjoy fruit, stick with 0 to 3 low-fructose fresh or frozen servings per day. If you can do without fruits, fine. In fact, if you are trying to lose 50 pounds or more, it is a good idea to skip fruit completely. There is no biological reason to eat fruit as long as you are consuming enough non-starchy vegetables. There's nothing essential in fruits that you cannot get, and with a lot less sugar, from NSVs.

A serving of a piece of fresh fruit is roughly the size of your fist. Other measurements include:

6 strawberries	½ cup of berries
1 orange	¼ melon
1 apricot	1 tablespoon of powdered
½ grapefruit	superfruits

SANE FOOD COMBINATIONS

For many people, eating nothing more than a cup of berries or a handful of cashews just makes them want more berries and cashews. This can lead to hunger. Eating an optimal amount of nuts and low-fructose fruits is easier if you combine them with NSVs and nutrient-dense protein.

The best way to do this is to think of whole-food fats and low-fructose fruits as scrumptious SANE desserts, and there are plenty of them in the recipe section. You can use nuts, nut flours, seeds, seed flours, cocoa/cacao, coconut, and berries to make SANE cookies, fudges, pies, cakes, ice cream, milkshakes, and other SANE treats that will satisfy any sweet tooth after an NSV and nutrient-dense, protein-rich meal.

Another critical point to remember: Studies show that you are more likely to lower your setpoint if you favor whole-food fats over low-fructose fruits. If you are extremely clogged, even the small amount of sugar in berries and citrus can slow your setpoint-lowering efforts. You can make surprising changes in your body, especially at the beginning of your journey, by limiting even low-fructose fruits.

Before we can wrap up our conversation about sweets, we've got to cover added sweeteners. It seems like every other day, food corporations come up with a new name for these setpoint-elevating monstrosities. For example, all of the following are basically sugar, from your setpoint's perspective:

Agave nectar

Barley malt

Beet sugar

Brown sugar

Buttered syrup

Cane crystals

Cane juice crystals

Cane sugar

Caramel

Carob syrup

Castor sugar

Confectioner's sugar

Corn sweetener

Corn syrup

Corn syrup solids

Crystalline fructose

Date sugar

Demerara sugar

Dextran

Dextrose

Diastatic malt

Diastase

Ethyl maltol

Evaporated cane juice

Fructose

Fruit juice

Fruit juice concentrates

Galactose

Glucose

Glucose solids

Golden sugar

Golden syrup

Granulated sugar

Grape sugar

High-fructose corn syrup

Honey

Icing sugar

Invert sugar

Lactose

Malt syrup

Maltodextrin

Maltose

Maple syrup

Molasses

Muscovado sugar

Panocha

Raw sugar

Refiner's syrup

Rice syrup

Sorbitol

Sorghum syrup

Sucrose

Sugar

Syrup

Treacle

Turbinado sugar

Yellow sugar

Memorizing this list isn't important. It is important to know that any form of caloric sweetener—other than the four safe sweeteners we'll cover in a moment—increases your setpoint. Your body does not care where sugar and sweetener calories come from. It's also important that you protect yourself from misleading "natural" marketing. *Unnatural* high-fructose corn syrup is 42 percent fructose. *Natural* agave nectar is about 90 percent fructose. Tobacco is also natural.

When it comes to sweets, I eat them daily, and you can eat them daily, too, while lowering your setpoint. All you have to do is practice "safe sweeteners." You do this simply by focusing on four fantastic and all-natural options: stevia, luo han guo (monk fruit), erythritol, and xylitol. The first two are natural herbs with a sweet taste. The last two are sugar alcohols found in fruits. None of them elevate your setpoint or do anything harmful to you as long as you enjoy them in their pure form. Most of what you will find on store shelves has a tiny bit of one of those four along with a bunch of inSANEity. We can help you find pure sources at SANESolution.com.

In terms of which to use when, if you are baking, use xylitol because it cooks like sugar. For everything else, use erythritol unless you already like stevia and luo han guo. Stevia and luo han guo are great, but most people find them hard to use, as they don't work, look, or taste anything like sugar. We'll cover this more in the cooking chapters, but by using these safe sweeteners and other SANE substitutions, you can "SANEitize" all of your favorite foods and never feel deprived while lowering your setpoint. You can have your cake and eat it, too (as long as you swap the sugar and flour out for SANE substitutes)!

SANE Points

- Every flavor can be enjoyed in abundance while going SANE.
- Getting most of your calories from whole-food fats makes your body good at burning fat as fuel. That makes weight loss much easier.
- Whole-food fats are essential for lowering your setpoint; low-fructose fruits are not.
- Avoid unnatural processed fats (most oils) completely; if needed, use stable, natural processed fats such as coconut oil for cooking.
- Pair whole-food fats or low-fructose fruits with non-starchy vegetables and nutrient-dense protein whenever possible.
- Whole-food fats and low-fructose fruits are SANE dessert superstars.
- If you really struggle with your weight, you will be likely to have better setpoint-lowering results if you focus more on whole-food fats instead of low-fructose fruits.
- If you need to add sweetness, use stevia, luo han guo, erythritol, and xylitol.

CHAPTER 7

Smoothies and Beverages

If you asked me, "Jonathan, if I could do only one thing to reach a lower setpoint, what would that be?" I'd immediately and unequivocally recommend that you get your blender out, make a SANE smoothie, and savor every sip!

A smoothie! Really? Yes! Before you raise your eyebrow, SANE smoothies are radically different from the sugar-saturated smoothies you find on grocery store shelves, health food stores, or at smoothie chains. The amount of sugar in those "healthy" smoothies makes cans of Mountain Dew blush.

SANE smoothies, on the other hand, contain less sugar than a handful of baby carrots. They have no artificial sweeteners nor unnatural chemicals or flavorings, are 100 percent gluten free, and your kids will love them—not to mention they may be the simplest and most setpoint-lowering breakfast, quick lunch, or snack imaginable.

On the Setpoint Diet, the SANE smoothie is a scrumptious green-vegetable-based drink that mainlines the most therapeutic setpoint-lowering nutrients possible into your body, deliciously and practically. It is the easiest way to take in as many optimal non-starchy vegetables as you can, while boosting your protein, vitamin, mineral, antioxidant, and fiber intake with the pulse of a blender. It is also one of the easiest and most beneficial ways you can transform your setpoint and your life.

SANE green smoothies are the closest thing to a "magic pill" there will ever be for lowering your setpoint, helping your body burn fat optimally, and more. Simply by adding one to three SANE smoothies to your daily meal plan, you will:

- Lower your setpoint.
- Lose weight.

- Unclog hormones.
- Accelerate your metabolism.
- Stay naturally thin—permanently.
- Heal your gut.
- Reduce neuroinflammation.
- Maximize Satiety, nonAggression, Nutrition, and inEfficiency.
- Control diabetes and diabesity.
- End overeating and cravings.
- Minimize cellulite.
- Develop lean muscle tissue.
- Enhance athletic performance.
- Improve all aspects of your health.

Ready to raise your glass?

SANE SMOOTHIES 101: TWO TRANSFORMATIVE TYPES

First, some general guidelines on SANE smoothies:

- A SANE smoothie will taste good enough—and better over time—but not like the liquid-candy smoothies sold at grocery stores and smoothie shops. That's a good thing.
- As you get used to green smoothies, start with spinach or romaine lettuce; these are less bitter than many other green, leafy vegetables.
- The more flexible or tender the green leafy vegetable, the better it will blend into a smoothie (very important if you do not have a high-powered blender).
- Focus on ease and simplicity when measuring serving sizes. A serving of raw spinach is what you can easily fit into your two hands cupped together. As a result, the serving size will vary from person to person.
- Ask yourself, "What is my purpose in making this smoothie? Will it be a snack or a meal?" This question—and its answer—will help you determine what goes into your smoothie.
- There is no one "right" formulation for a smoothie..

- Do what you want your children to do. Your kids may not want to drink green smoothies right away, but the more they see you enjoying them, the more they'll want some too. Green smoothies are a great way to get your kids enjoying lots of veggies.
- The first time you try something bitter, you may not like it because bitter is an acquired taste (e.g., wine and beer). As you continue to drink smoothies, however, they will taste delicious, and you'll acquire healthy cravings for them.
- A green smoothie is the single most concentrated source of real food nutrition you can take in and is a great way to heal your body from a variety of ailments.

On the Setpoint Diet, you maximize your results by enjoying two types of SANE smoothies in order to flip your metabolism into fat-burning mode and get closer to your ideal setpoint: the SANE All-Veggie Smoothie and the SANE Meal Smoothie.

The SANE All-Veggie Smoothie

The *only* goal of the All-Veggie Smoothie is to easily increase your optimal non-starchy vegetable intake so that you begin to lower your setpoint right away. All-Veggie Smoothies can also be enjoyed throughout the day to help you easily increase your vegetable intake, and support and accelerate fat-burning. The All-Veggie Smoothie is also the perfect complement to a meal that already contains protein and whole-food fats. For example, you can enjoy one of these smoothies at breakfast, along with a plate of scrambled egg whites and whole eggs. This makes a complete SANE breakfast (non-starchy vegetables, nutrient-dense proteins, and whole-food fats).

The SANE Meal Smoothie

The SANE Meal Smoothie is designed to be used as a meal, because unlike the All-Veggie Smoothie, it contains nutrient-dense protein. This smoothie is perfect if you don't have time to cook.

This is important: Because the SANE Meal Smoothies serve as your entire meal, they should contain:

- 2 to 5 servings of green non-starchy vegetables.
- 1 to 2 servings of nutrient-dense proteins (see below). Ideal nutrient-dense protein for SANE smoothies includes clean

whey protein concentrate, pasteurized egg whites, or unflavored Greek yogurt. If you are a vegan or vegetarian, clean pea protein concentrate is a good alternative to whey protein. The right quantity and quality of protein can turn you into a slim and strong fat-burning machine.

- Optional whole-food fats (1 to 2 servings) such as ⅛ cup of unsweetened shredded coconut, raw undutched cocoa, chia seeds, flax seeds, or a slice or two of avocado.

(Please note: The All-Veggie Smoothies do not contain proteins or whole-food fats—just lots of green veggies and a little bit of low-fructose fruits!)

SANE SMOOTHIE INGREDIENTS

To create SANE smoothies, I advise taking a simple paint-by-numbers approach, in which your blender is your canvas and you have five "colors" to work with:

1. Non-starchy vegetables. These include primarily greens, such as spinach, kale, or romaine lettuce; cucumbers; celery; and so forth.

Start with a base of a cup of water and add two big handfuls of spinach and two big handfuls of romaine lettuce to your blender. Both types of greens are less bitter than many other green, leafy vegetables. It's fine to use frozen varieties of greens, too, but keep in mind, spinach is available in frozen form, whereas romaine lettuce is not, because it doesn't freeze well. (Try experimenting with other greens such as kale or arugula once you master the basics.)

As you experiment more with your green smoothies, you'll discover other non-starchy vegetable combinations that yield even more nutrition in a quick and portable smoothie than most people consume in a week. Green smoothies may seem scary at first, but after trying them for a week and seeing how you look and feel, you may find that living without them starts to feel even scarier.

2. Nutrient-dense proteins. If you're making a SANE Meal Smoothie, it should include a protein. Your body deserves the cleanest, most high-quality protein available, so select from one of the following:

Clean whey protein or a vegetable-based protein powder. This is the ideal protein for your smoothies. The only catch is that you must avoid unnatural whey products containing flavoring, sweeteners, and fillers. If the ingredients contain anything other than whey proteins, skip it because those additives can cause weight gain. (For more information on the power of whey to help lower your setpoint, see Chapter 10.) If you are a vegan or a vegetarian, use clean pea protein concentrate.

Pasteurized egg whites. These are 90 percent protein and are sold in ready-to-use containers at most grocery stores. Make sure they are pasteurized so they are safe to add directly (without cooking) to your smoothies.

Unflavored nonfat Greek yogurt. This is not your optimal choice but still SANE, Greek yogurt contains 67 percent protein. Use it for variety and a change of pace.

Whichever protein you pick from these choices, add enough so that smoothies contain at least 24 grams of protein but no more than 50 grams.

These proteins make the perfect SANE Meal Smoothie—no need to try blending tuna in the mix. I tried it once, and the results were, let's say, less than tasty.

3. SANE sweeteners. These sweeteners are 100 percent natural—no damaging doses of refined, setpoint-elevating sugar at all—but deliciously sweet anyway. Choose from the following:

Oranges. Low in sugar and high in flavor and vitamins, half a peeled orange sweetens smoothies, amazingly and deliciously, especially in smoothies packed with green vegetables.

Frozen strawberries. Convenient and inexpensive, a handful of these frozen berries provides a low sugar and high-nutrition sweet boost to smoothies. Note: You can use any frozen berries, but strawberries seem to offer the best taste and texture.

As a general rule of thumb, all berries and citrus are low-fructose fruits, so those are what you want to focus on, while keeping in mind that if you have more than 50 pounds to lose, I recommend that you stay away from all fruit except for lemons, avocados, and tomatoes (yes . . . avocados and tomatoes are fruits), at least until you reach your goal weight.

Natural noncalorie sugar substitute erythritol. Found in many fruits, erythritol adds zero-calorie sweetness to anything without harming blood sugar or causing tooth decay. It's an ideal option if you want sweetness without fruit flavor or would like to minimize your sugar intake. This sweetener also pairs well with oranges and strawberries. Start with a teaspoon and sweeten to your taste preference.

4. Superfood enhancers. One easy way to get optimal nutrition from whole foods (particularly if you have a busy schedule) is to supplement your smoothies with powdered "superfoods." With all the convenience of a vitamin pill, plus all the high-quality and natural-context benefits of whole foods, superfoods are a concentrated source of vitamins, minerals, enzymes, antioxidants, fiber, and essential amino acids. They can give you incredible energy, fend off disease, and even accelerate your body's fat-burning powers.

Available at most health food stores, superfood enhancers include non-starchy vegetable powders such as wheatgrass, spirulina, moringa, or combinations of these ingredients. A tablespoon or two will supercharge your smoothie and further increase your daily serving of non-starchy vegetables. A whole lot more information on these is available at SANESolution.com.

5. Taste turbochargers. These natural, healing ingredients have special powers over appetite, blood sugar control, gut health, and inflammation—all factors that lower your setpoint:

Raw undistilled apple cider vinegar. This turbocharger has been clinically shown to improve insulin sensitivity and blood sugar. This means that it bolsters insulin's ability to bring sugar out of the bloodstream and into the cells of the body. Research shows that it can slow blood sugar response (unhealthy hikes in glucose) by as much as 34 percent.

This is not its only benefit, however. Apple cider vinegar has been correlated with reduced belly fat, slimmer waist circumference, lower blood triglycerides, and weight loss.

You don't need much, either—just a half teaspoon for every handful of green veggies added to your smoothie. It not only accents the taste of green leafy vegetables in your smoothie, it also helps your body digest those veggies so you don't have to worry about bloating or gas. The only catch is that just not any vinegar will work. You must use the raw, undistilled, unfiltered variety—available from online retailers such as Amazon or in the "healthy" section of most grocery stores.

Lemons. With just a single gram of sugar, plenty of vitamin C, and well-known detox and digestion benefits, lemons offer the unique ability to eliminate the bitterness from green leafy vegetables. Cut the peel off your lemon and toss into the blender with your other ingredients.

Guar gum. Derived from the guar bean, this special fiber has eight times the thickening power of cornstarch and adds another level of smoothness to smoothies. Guar gum has been clinically studied for its benefits on several conditions affecting setpoint. This fiber:

- Reduces blood glucose and thus improves glycemic control.
- Promotes healthy gut bacteria (guar gum is a prebiotic, feeding the probiotic bacteria in the gastrointestinal tract and providing them with a better environment in which to thrive).
- Reduces neuroinflammation.
- Curbs cravings and prevents overeating.
- Supports heart health by reducing blood pressure and improving cholesterol profiles.

Add ⅛ teaspoon of guar gum to your smoothie, and continue adding ⅛ teaspoon until the desired consistency is reached. A little goes a long way.

Konjac root. Also called konjac glucomannan, konjac root powder helps create a deliciously smooth texture in your smoothies. As a fiber, it creates a feeling of fullness, too. Konjac:

- Is a prebiotic that feeds the friendly bacteria in your gut.
- Helps balance your blood sugar.
- Has been shown to help normalize cholesterol.

Add ⅛ teaspoon of konjac to your smoothie, and continue adding ⅛ teaspoon until the desired consistency is reached.

Cinnamon. You may have some cinnamon sitting in your spice rack. Now you'll want to use a lot more of it immediately in your smoothies. For thousands of years, cinnamon has been prized for its many remarkable medicinal properties and is one of our best-loved spices. Cinnamon is also a great way to pump up the flavor and sweetness of your smoothie without adding extra sweeteners like honey or sugar. Cinnamon:

- Can dramatically reduce insulin resistance and lower blood sugar levels.
- Ranks #1 out of 26 spices studied for antioxidant activity. (The antioxidants in cinnamon heal inflammation.)
- Helps reduce levels of bad cholesterol, while increasing good cholesterol.
- Interferes with the formation of a protein called tau in the brain, which is one of the hallmarks of Alzheimer's disease.

Add ¼ teaspoon of cinnamon for every two handfuls of green veggies in your smoothie—up to 1 teaspoon daily.

Gelatin. I bet you've eaten Jell-O. I can't wait for you to try its close—but super-healthier—cousin: unflavored gelatin. To make sure you flip your metabolism into fat-burning mode, put gelatin into as many of your smoothies as possible. In addition to making them much more satisfying, unflavored gelatin is a clean source of otherwise hard-to-find nutrients that offer several benefits. Gelatin:

- Makes your skin glow by suppling glycine and proline, two amino acids that are used in the production of collagen (a protein that gives skin its firmness).
- Reduces joint pain, again thanks to glycine and proline and their ability to stimulate collagen production, which acts as a natural fire extinguisher for joint pain.
- Helps you sleep (quality sleep is important to helping you achieve a lower setpoint. Glycine is also an inhibitory neurotransmitter, which can decrease anxiety while promoting calmness and sleep quality).
- Heals your gut—also critical in setpoint lowering. Gelatin effectively enhances gastric acid secretion for better digestion and restores a healthy stomach lining.
- Helps support your metabolism so that your body can switch into fat-burning mode.

Add ½ to 1 teaspoon of gelatin per cup of your smoothie.

SANE SMOOTHIE ORDER OF OPERATIONS

If you don't have one already, invest in a quality blender. The one I recommend is a reconditioned Vitamix. It's what the professionals use, and if you get it reconditioned you'll save a lot of money. You can get a special discount and free shipping at SANESolution.com. The difference between a Vitamix and a conventional blender is like the difference between an airplane and a car. One is much faster and gets you to places the other just can't. If you plan on making smoothies every day, as this plan recommends, treat yourself to a Vitamix. (I'm not here to be a salesperson, so let me just say that I've used my Vitamix daily for 10 years. I love it.)

1. Pour in the liquid (a cup of water is recommended). Start with a ¼ cup of water per handful of vegetables, and adjust to your desired consistency.

2. Add your green leafy vegetables. Without touching the blender blades, pack in as many green veggies as you can into the base of the blender.

3. Add everything else: protein and *optional* whole-food fats (if making a SANE Meal Smoothie), SANE sweeteners, superfoods, and turbochargers.

4. Put the blender lid on. Sounds obvious, but it takes forgetting once to know that it's worth adding to the order of operations.

5. Blend the smoothie for up to 3 minutes. This ensures that you have the smoothest smoothie possible—no grainy chunks, just a delicious milkshake-like consistency. In fact, you want the smoothie to be warm (from the friction of the blender blades) before you turn off the blender. This is another way to ensure the smoothness of your smoothie. If you are going to drink your smoothie right away, add some crushed iced to make sure it's nice and cold. If you're going to drink it later, simply refrigerate it, and reblend for a nice refreshing smoothie.

If you'd like to see SANE smoothie-making in action, view the videos at SANESolution.com.

Savory Smoothies—AKA Soups!

Here's a delicious twist on the SANE smoothie: Take a mixture of veggies (frozen is very convenient!) like broccoli, cauliflower, carrots, and tomatoes, and blend them in 1 or 2 cups of water or MSG-free broth. Add some garlic and your favorite seasonings, and maybe some whole-food fats. Blend for longer than 3 minutes—until the mixture is warm. Pour it into a bowl. Voila—You just took all your new smoothie magic and transformed it into a tasty vegetable soup. If you have any leftover cooked poultry, stir it in, and you've now punched up the protein for a super-SANE, super-satiating meal. (There are more SANE soup recipes in Appendix A.)

The SANE Smoothie Batch Blending Plan

To save time and be even more successful, make more than one smoothie at a time. In fact, to save the most time, batch blend all your SANE smoothie for the week at once. Here's how it works:

1. The day you're going to "batch blend," head to the grocery store and purchase all the produce you need for that week.
2. Prep all the produce.
3. Blend your smoothies as directed in the order of operations.
4. Place all your smoothies in any sort of plastic container, shaker bottle, or reused Greek yogurt container that you have on hand.
5. Put 4 days' worth of smoothies in your refrigerator; and 3 days in your freezer.
6. When you take a smoothie out of the refrigerator, replace it with one from the freezer.
7. Reblend each smoothie prior to drinking it.

OTHER SANE FLUIDS

When your body is well hydrated, it starts decreasing the concentration of various substances in the blood, and this turbocharges fat-burning. Additionally, adequate hydration provides a feeling of Satiety and tends to fill you up, making it much easier to avoid inSANE setpoint-elevating processed foods and sugary drinks. Your heart, liver, lungs, skin—every organ, down to every single cell—love being hydrated and will reward you for it—with a slim, energized body.

In addition to your setpoint-lowering SANE smoothies, hydrate your body with these options:

Green Tea

Fall in love with green tea. It comes from the same plant as black tea (the tea most common in the United States and Europe), but it is processed differently.

Its unique processing leaves green tea with a large amount of substances called *polyphenols*—especially EGCG (epigallocatechin gallate)—that assist the body in burning fat and reducing insulin resistance. Researchers suspect green tea's unique fat-burning effect has to do with the interaction of this tea's polyphenols, caffeine, and the hormone noradrenaline.

To maximize all the benefits green tea has to offer, it's helpful to drink a lot of it daily—at least 10 bags' worth. I know what you're thinking: "Ten bags of green tea on top of all that water? I'm going to spend all day in the bathroom, and I'll be really jittery."

Not to worry. If you drink ten 8-ounce cups of green tea, that counts as ten 8-ounce cups of water. Also, you can brew eight bags of green tea at a time in 12 ounces of water. Let it sit for a few minutes, add ice, and then drink it quickly. Do that once in the morning and once in the afternoon and you have easily and effortlessly consumed an optimal amount of setpoint-lowering polyphenols.

Compared to a cup of brewed coffee, which can contain up to 150 milligrams of caffeine, green tea is pretty low in caffeine—at 30 milligrams in one tea bag. Ten bags of green tea deliver roughly the same amount of caffeine to your body as 2 cups of coffee. If you don't want the caffeine, choose decaf green tea. It's as healthy and helpful as regular green tea. It's perfectly fine to drink black or white tea, too, if that's your preference. All three teas come from the same plant. Either way, enjoy!

Kombucha Tea

Try kombucha tea as an alternative. This fermented drink contains gut-healing probiotics or "good bacteria" and therefore is helpful in lowering your setpoint.

A word of important advice about kombucha tea: Many products are high in sugar. If you're interested in adding kombucha, check the labels. Select only products that contain less than 6 grams of sugar per 12 ounces.

Water

Your body requires at least 8 8-ounce glasses of water per day to burn body fat effectively—and you'll probably get up to three of those glasses from your daily SANE smoothies. More fluid is always better.

To make it easy to enjoy over 8 glasses of water per day, try these tips:

- The easiest way to drink an optimal amount of water is to fill up a gallon (128-ounce) jug in the morning and to make sure it is empty 2 hours before you go to bed.
- Drink your water cold. Continuously drinking cold water raises your metabolic rate. Studies show you burn about 2 additional calories for every ounce of cold water you drink. Cold water also slows down the emptying of food from your stomach. Because the water hangs around longer, it gives your hunger hormones time to tell your brain that you're hydrated.

SANE Vitamin Water

Don't like plain water? Make your own SANE "vitamin water." Fill your blender three-quarters full with water. Add two frozen strawberries or a slice of orange. Add ⅛ teaspoon of guar gum and a handful of ice. Add SANE sweeteners if you'd like. Blend for 1 minute. Pour the mixture into reusable bottles and refrigerate or freeze. There you have it—delicious vitamin- and fiber-packed water that's ready to go. Play around with other natural flavors such as sliced cucumber, fresh mint, and lime, and make your own signature flavor.

Pumping up your hydration from any of these SANE fluids makes it easier to avoid sugary beverages—which are leading us down the path to obesity and chronic diseases instead of good health. A California Center for Public Health Advocacy study found that adults who drink one or more sodas per day were 27 percent more apt to be overweight or obese compared with those who do not drink soda.

So for fluids, go SANE. If it is a SANE smoothie, water, green tea, or kombucha, drinking a sufficient amount will help you get to a lower setpoint fast and furiously.

SANE Points

- Adequate hydration is extremely important for lowering your setpoint, encouraging fat-burning, healing your metabolism, and building optimal health.
- Enjoy one to three SANE smoothies per day as part of your meal plan. They are the closest thing to a "magic pill" there will ever be for lowering setpoint and more—and the easiest way to consume double-digit servings of raw non-starchy vegetables daily.
- Drink over 64 ounces of SANE fluid daily. In addition to your one to three SANE smoothies daily, choose from green tea, water, SANE vitamin water, or kombucha.

PART 3

SANE MEALS, COOKING, AND NUTRACEUTICALS

CHAPTER 8

Meal Planning for a Lower Setpoint

Now comes what most people consider the fun part (I'm a science guy, but cooking can be fun, too)! You're ready to get down to the essence of planning SANE meals—and how they work as a lifelong, enjoyable, simple, and delicious way of eating.

Imagine that you've invited friends to your home for dinner. You serve them a feast of tossed green salad, roasted butternut squash, mashed cauliflower, a scrumptious grilled roast beef, flax bread, and a beautiful cheesecake for dessert. Each of these dishes can be made SANEly, although they seem like delicious indulgences. None of your guests would ever believe that you've just served them a healthy, setpoint-lowering meal—one in which no one has to worry about calories or trying to burn or starve them off the next day. Yet this is life when you are SANE. And the feast you just served? It's an example of what SANE meal planning looks like.

What it doesn't look like is the typical patronizing, eat-exactly-this series of menus. You see a lot of diets try to tell you exactly what to eat at every meal. If you encounter a diet like that, run the other way.

How realistic is it for someone who knows nothing about you to tell you exactly what to eat for every meal of every day? We all have different tastes, allergies, intolerances, and preferences in food. A plan blindly telling you to "eat exactly this" next week (all the way down to portion size) works about as well as a plan telling you to "wear exactly this" next week (all the way down to pants or dress size). What if you are going to a wedding? What if you are going to the beach? How can a plan know what will fit with your unique life without knowing you personally? It can't, and these sorts of diet plans stop working the minute life happens. But don't worry, you are done with that ineffective approach. SANE eating forever frees you from hard-and-fast menu rules and confusing and conflicting weight-loss information you've been told before.

SANE empowers you to plan your own meals that satisfy your likes and desires. While you will be given some specific guidelines to get you started on the first 21 days, think of these guidelines like training wheels: You start off with training wheels, but as soon as you learn to ride and build your confidence, they come off. Before long, meal planning will become second nature, and you'll be able to eat SANEly for a lifetime.

Lifetime is the key word here. Any wellness or dietary program that you can't keep up forever will never give you the long-lasting results you deserve and will actually harm your health. A 7-day cleanse may sound tantalizing, but what happens on day 8? With this plan, you'll get focused on the next 30 years and beyond...not just the next 30 days or less.

Before you get started, let's quickly review the number of servings of SANE foods to eat daily.

Non-starchy vegetables: 10+ servings daily
Nutrient-dense protein: 100 to 200 grams daily (in 25-gram to 50-gram
    doses)
Whole-food fats: 1 to 6 servings daily
Low-fructose fruits: 0 to 3 servings daily

The more SANE foods you eat, the more you'll want to eat them every single day and will feel their power at work all day long. As for cravings—like longing to wolf down a box of cookies or getting up close and personal with a bag of chips—they'll disappear.

The modern science of health and fitness has revealed that as frustrating as cravings are, we can rewire ourselves to crave healthier foods. In a 2000 study published in *Physiology & Behavior*, researchers instructed subjects to consume a diet of what most people would consider a very unappealing nutritional drink for 1 week (Pelchat and Schaefer 2000). But after the experimental period ended, several participants reported craving that drink later—a finding that surprised the researchers.

Or here's another example you may have personal experience with. Did you enjoy dry red wine the first time you tried it? Do you enjoy it now? If you are like many people, something that was unappealing became delicious and crave-worthy after you got used to it. Now imagine if setpoint-lowering foods worked that way. Good news: They do!

When you eat SANE foods, you harness the power of a part of your brain called the *orbitofrontal cortex* to rewire your cravings. Through a process known as *neuroplasticity*, when you consistently eat SANEly, your orbitofrontal cortex, along with other parts of your brain, physically change and reprogram you to crave setpoint-lowering foods as deeply as you may currently crave setpoint-elevating foods. As Peter Vishton, PhD, associate professor of psychology at William & Mary, notes: "Pleasure isn't in the food, it's in your head," and that's great, because it means you can rewire your brain to crave SANE. I know it sounds too good to be true, but it's proven science. You can crave non-starchy vegetables while finding soda disgusting. It's all about your brain wiring, and upgrading that wiring is exactly what your 21-Day Plan will do.

This is one of the key reasons SANE eating works long-term: The more SANE food you eat, the more you will like the taste of SANE food. SANE foods taste great, make you feel completely full and satisfied, heal your hormones, lower your setpoint, and ignite your body's natural fat-burning power. You'll be empowered to make this happen with help from the delicious meal recipes in Appendix A, and from the 1,600-plus recipes at SANESolution.com—so be sure to check them out and adopt some new family favorites.

YOUR SANE PLATE

An important and simple tool for meal planning is the SANE Plate, an intuitive, visual way to create balanced, SANE meals. It takes all the craziness out of figuring out what to eat, planning, shopping, and thinking about all of that. Like you did in creating your SANE smoothies, you'll take a paint-by-numbers approach to meal planning to fill your SANE Plate at breakfast, lunch, and dinner. It really is the easiest way to lower your setpoint and start seeing the results you want.

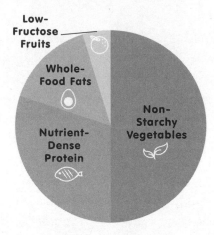

Here's how to design your plate at each meal and create the right SANE mix to automatically start lowering your setpoint and burn fat.

Step 1

Fill half your SANE Plate with non-starchy vegetables, such as spinach, kale, romaine lettuce, broccoli, mushrooms, peppers, asparagus—any veggie you could eat raw. Put the emphasis on green leafy vegetables as much as possible.

Step 2

Fill one-third of your SANE Plate with nutrient-dense protein. Great sources of protein include seafood, shellfish, poultry, beef, nonfat Greek yogurt, and nonfat cottage cheese. When protein takes up one-third of your plate, about the size of your hand, you easily obtain the 25 to 50 grams you need at each meal without obsessive measuring or weighing.

Step 3

Fill the remainder of your plate with whole-food fats. Remember, therapeutic fats found in foods such as avocados, nuts, olives, coconuts, eggs, and cocoa are scientifically proven to burn fat.

As for low-fructose fruits, these are an optional add-on to the SANE food groups. You can enjoy up to 1 to 3 servings daily of low-fructose fruits, such as berries and citrus. Again, if your long-term goals include lowering your setpoint weight by more than 50 pounds, you should stay away from all fruit (except for lemons) until you reach your goal weight.

SANE MEALS

Let's look at some examples of real-life SANE Plates, with typical SANE foods and serving estimations for what you'll be eating. Please note that the serving sizes are intentional approximations and general guidelines. It's easy to overcomplicate things in talking about servings and serving sizes. I don't want you to get caught up in measuring every single serving—please don't sweat the small stuff. Stay focused on the big picture and estimate your intake as accurately as you can. The SANE Plate proportions will keep you automatically on track, without having to use scales or other measuring devices.

Meals like those below are designed to ensure you get SANE, balanced, healthy meals every time you eat—meals with the proper amount of nutrient-dense proteins, non-starchy vegetables, and whole-food fats. Remember, too, that for best results, and to easily get in your quota of non-starchy veggies, enjoy one to three SANE smoothies daily, punched up with *optimal* NSVs, superfood powders, or both.

Sample SANE Breakfasts

SANE Veggie Scramble: 2 eggs and 3 egg whites, scrambled with a lot of non-starchy veggies (two big handfuls of green and red bell pepper and one handful of onion)

SANE translation: 1 nutrient-dense protein, 3 non-starchy vegetables, 1 whole-food fat (2 eggs = 12 grams protein; 3 egg whites = 12 grams protein; ¼ cup diced ham = 8 grams protein. This totals 32 grams protein, which equates to 1 serving of nutrient-dense protein).

SANE Meal Smoothie for Breakfast

SANE translation: 1 nutrient-dense protein, 3 NSVs, 1 whole-food fat (2 scoops clean whey protein = 36 grams protein, which equates to 1 serving of nutrient-dense protein).

SANE Spinach and Mushroom Omelet: 2 eggs and 4 egg whites with a filling of mushrooms and spinach (about 1 cup cooked)

SANE translation: 1 nutrient-dense protein, 3 NSVs, 1 whole-food fat (2 eggs = 12 grams protein; 4 egg whites = 16 grams protein. This totals 28 grams protein, which roughly equates to 1 serving of nutrient-dense protein).

Smoked salmon, served with capers, lettuce leaves, sliced red onion, sliced tomato, and avocado slices

SANE translation: 1 nutrient-dense protein, 3 NSVs, 1 whole-food fat (4.5 ounces salmon = 30 grams protein, which equates to 1 serving of nutrient-dense protein).

Grain-free cereal (1 tablespoon each of chopped cashews, almonds, hazelnuts, shredded coconut, and flaxseeds or chia seeds) mixed with about 1 cup of nonfat Greek yogurt or cottage cheese

SANE translation: 1 nutrient-dense protein, 2 whole-food fats (1 cup nonfat Greek yogurt or cottage cheese = 25 to 28 grams protein, which equates to 1 serving of nutrient-dense protein).

Sample SANE Lunches

Stir-fry chicken with lots of NSVs (use just enough coconut or avocado oil needed to prevent sticking, or stir-fry with broth or water)

SANE translation: 1 nutrient-dense protein, 3 NSVs (one 6-ounce chicken breast = 39 grams protein, which equates to 1 serving of nutrient-dense protein).

Greek-style salad: Large green salad with sliced cucumber, onion, and bell pepper; olives; and roasted chicken breast, dressed with a mixture of red wine vinegar, salt, pepper, and Greek yogurt

SANE translation: 1 nutrient-dense protein, 3 NSVs, 1 whole-food fat (one 6-ounce chicken breast = 39 grams protein, which equates to 1 serving of nutrient-dense protein).

Garden fruit salad: Large bed of romaine lettuce, 1 cup of cottage cheese, topped with walnuts and your favorite berries

SANE translation: 1 nutrient-dense protein, 3 NSVs, 1 whole-food fat, 1 low-fructose fruit (1 cup nonfat cottage cheese = 28 grams protein, which equals 1 serving of nutrient-dense protein).

Tuna salad lettuce wraps: Several large leaves of romaine lettuce filled with tuna, mixed with some chopped onions, tomatoes, and several chopped olives

SANE translation: 1 nutrient-dense protein, 3 NSVs, 1 whole-food fat (1 cup tuna = 39 grams protein, which equates to 1 serving of nutrient-dense protein).

SANE hummus and chicken: Make SANE hummus using steamed cauliflower instead of chickpeas, lemon, cumin, coriander, and 1 tablespoon of tahini; skip the olive oil. Scoop up the SANE hummus with raw vegetables like tomatoes, cucumbers, bell peppers, and lettuce and grilled chicken.

SANE translation: 1 nutrient-dense protein, 3 NSVs, 1 whole-food fat (one 6-ounce chicken breast = 39 grams protein, which equates to 1 serving of nutrient-dense protein).

Sample SANE Dinners

Generous fillet of baked white fish crusted with sliced almonds (or other nut crust), grilled non-starchy vegetables

SANE translation: 1 nutrient-dense protein, 3 NSVs, 1 whole-food fat (one 6-ounce piece of white fish = 45 grams protein, which equates to 1 serving of nutrient-dense protein).

Grilled grass-fed sirloin steak with Green Beans Almondine (green beans sautéed with slivered almonds) and mashed cauliflower

SANE translation: 1.5 nutrient-dense proteins, 3 NSVs, 1 whole-food fat (one 5-ounce steak = 43 grams protein, which equates to 1 serving of nutrient-dense protein).

Baked salmon fillet over a bed of riced cauliflower

SANE translation: 1 nutrient-dense protein, 3 NSVs, 1 whole-food fat (one 6-ounce salmon fillet = 38 grams protein, which equates to 1 serving of nutrient-dense protein).

Several slices of pork tenderloin, with a walnut and red cabbage slaw
    SANE translation: 1 nutrient-dense protein, 3 NSVs, 1 whole-food fat (one 5-ounce slice of pork tenderloin = 40 grams protein, which equates to 1 serving of nutrient-dense protein).

Lean ground beef or turkey, cooked with diced tomato, green peppers, onions, and taco seasonings, served in several large leaves of romaine lettuce, with a few avocado slices or guacamole
    SANE translation: 1 nutrient-dense protein, 3 NSVs, 1 whole-food fat (one 5-ounce lean ground turkey or lean ground beef = 27 to 37 grams protein, which equates to 1 serving of nutrient-dense protein).

If you decide to create your own SANE meal combinations (and you will), just look to the SANE Plate for guidelines, and you really can't miss.

DELICIOUS SANE SUBSTITUTIONS FOR STARCHES AND SWEETS

Staying SANE isn't about deprivation. It's about enjoying so much good food that you're too full for the setpoint-elevating stuff. And you can stay SANE—while cooking and eating almost anything—by making some simple swaps. Any food can be "SANEitized." So can beverages. If you love soda, for example, you can still make a SANEer version of it: Blend half a peeled orange completely. Stir it into a glass of carbonated water and add SANE sweeteners (such as erythritol) to taste, and you've just created a delightful orange soda. I could fill a book with these, and have, at SANESolution.com, so be sure to check those out.

    SANE swaps do double duty, too: They are an easy and surprisingly tasty way to prepare all your setpoint-lowering food, while at the same time satisfying your cravings for sweets and starches. Although these swaps will taste slightly different, they will also make you look and feel completely different—a trade-off that you will very much enjoy long-term. The chart below will get you started on SANEly swapping your way to slimness. Use your creativity and have fun making your favorite meals SANE!

SANE Swaps

inSANE	SANE
Pasta and rice	• Spaghetti squash/Squoodles • Zucchini noodles/Zoodles • Shirataki noodles • Shredded cabbage • Shaved Brussels sprouts • Bean sprouts • Pea shoots • Cauliflower rice, parsnip rice • Broccoli and carrot slaw (premade in grocery produce section) Each of the above swaps can serve as a delicious "bed" for SANE tomato and other sauces, stir-fries, salsas, and more.
Potatoes	• Mashed cauliflower • Turnips or radishes • Eggplant • Squash • Zucchini
Bread and tortillas	• Flax, coconut flour, almond flour, and psyllium • Lettuce leaves, collard leaves, kale leaves (with the rib removed), wilted cabbage leaves, thin-sliced cucumbers, and nori are all excellent replacements for sandwich wraps and tortillas.
Cookies, cakes, pies	• Baked goods made using golden flaxseed meal, coconut flour, almond meal, and other nut flours (see recipes in Appendix A).
Sugar, honey, syrups, jam	• Erythritol, xylitol, monk fruit (lo han guo), low-fructose fruits, and vegetable glycerin
Hot and cold cereals	• SANE cereals made with cooked pumpkin, coconut, ground flax, nuts, and/or chia (see recipes in Appendix A).

inSANE	SANE
Pretzels and chips	• Raw nuts
	• Seeds
	• Baked kale chips
	• Baked pork rinds, raw veggies, and flaked coconut
	SANE Bake-N-Crisps
Candy bars, energy bars, energy drinks, snack packs	SANE Bars and Energy Bites
Sweet coffee beverages	Use unsweetened coconut or almond milk, raw undutched cocoa, any natural noncaloric flavoring, any SANE sweetener.
	Note: Coffee is fine while going SANE as long as you don't add inSANE things to it.
Cow's Milk	Unsweetened almond or coconut milk

SANE SNACKS

You'll find that you won't need to snack much because your meals will be full of Satiating food. As a general rule, if you need to snack, you're probably not eating enough SANE foods at mealtimes and should reassess the composition of those meals. But if you need a little energy boost or you're simply craving a sweet, salty, or crunchy treat, here are the top go-to options:

1. SANE All-Veggie Smoothies (See recipes in Appendix A.)
   This tops the list because it's vital for setpoint-lowering that you drink one to three SANE smoothies daily. All-Veggie Smoothies are the perfect snack because they supply you therapeutically with at least 3 servings of non-starchy veggies.
2. Hard- or soft-boiled eggs
3. Raw non-starchy vegetables (eaten plain or with salsa, hummus, or ranch dip made with nonfat Greek yogurt)
4. Low-sugar jerky or unprocessed lunch meats
5. Protein bars that contain at least 20 grams of high-quality and clean protein, at least 10 grams of prebiotic fiber, no added sugars, no gluten, no soy, and nothing artificial. More info at SANESolution.com

6. Berries and/or low-sugar clean protein powder mixed with plain nonfat Greek yogurt or cottage cheese

7. SANE treats, like fudge, cake, pie, cookies, pudding, or ice cream (See recipes in Appendix A.)

8. Baked kale chips

9. Olives

10. Pickles

11. Kimchi

12. Baked pork rinds

13. SANE Bake-N-Crisps

14. Nuts or seeds

15. Sugar-free drinks with as few chemicals in them as possible (ideally these would be sweetened with a natural noncaloric sweetener such as stevia)

SANE DESSERTS

SANE desserts are typically made with whole-food fats and/or nutrient-dense protein and/or low-fructose fruits sweetened with SANE sugar substitutes. Some of these are so SANE that you can use them as main components of a snack or even a meal, as long as you get your quota of non-starchy vegetables in daily. Most of our members find that SANE desserts are the best way to enjoy whole-food fats. They focus their meals on NSVs and nutrient-dense protein, and then love their whole-food fats in a SANE dessert. For example, plenty of grilled zucchini and eggplant, along with a grass-fed steak or salmon, followed up with SANE peanut butter fudge makes an amazing, dessert-included meal.

SANE MEALS FOR THE WHOLE FAMILY

Great news! No more making a separate meal for yourself while the rest of your family eats food they actually enjoy. SANE meals are family-friendly—on two levels. First, you and your entire family already eat and love a lot of SANE foods. There's likely, however, a good amount of inSANE food also in the mix. So your strategy is to simply eat so much of the SANE food that you are too full for the setpoint-elevating inSANEity.

On taco Tuesday, have taco shells and add a crispy romaine lettuce "shells" option. On spaghetti night, serve your favorite meat sauce over wheat pasta and also set a bowl of zoodles (zucchini noodles) out. We call this technique "modular meals," and it is great for gradually transitioning your family to SANE eating, or for situations when you need to cater to several different types of eaters. For more tips and ideas for modular meals, visit SANESolution.com.

Second, SANE meals are the healthiest way to eat for everyone in your family: children, teens, adults, older adults, and anyone else. Think about it like this: How could eating food that prevents overeating (Satiety) while optimizing your hormones (Aggression) and giving you the most nutrition per calorie (Nutrition) without packing on body fat (Efficiency) *not* be healthy for everyone?

One quick anecdote about how profoundly eating SANE can impact your health. For years, my wife and I postponed trying to start a family until I was 35 and she was 36. Our doctors told us that because of us both working over 70 hours per week, our age, and how long my wife was on hormonal birth control, it was very unlikely we'd be able to conceive regardless of how "healthy" we both claimed to be. We tried to get pregnant for the first time on November 26, 2017. We conceived our first child on November 27, 2017.

My wife and I 100 percent practice what we preach; we are #SANE4Life (which you'll learn more about in a few chapters). We were overjoyed that despite what all the doctors told us, our choice to be #SANE4Life seems to have enabled us to beat the odds for creating life. SANE eating is simply the best way to live, and possibly even the best way to create life.

Did my wife continue to eat SANE during her pregnancy? Absolutely. Providing optimal nutrition to children (whether in or out of the womb) is nothing short of a moral imperative considering what's happening with the childhood obesity epidemic. SANE is not only fine for children, but it's even *more* important for children as well. When we feed our kids (or grandkids, nieces, nephews, or any little ones we care for) SANEly, we:

Give them the abundant nutrition their growing bodies need. Your kids require more nutrition than you do. Water-, fiber-, and protein-rich SANE foods contain more nutrition per calorie than any other foods, making this plan ideal for your children. They are still growing, so they need optimal nutrition from the most essential vitamins, minerals, proteins, and fats possible. There is no richer source of these than SANE meals.

Give them calories without giving them prediabetes, weight problems, or heart disease. Growing children need a lot of calories. In the traditional Western diet, these calories come from sugars, starches, and processed fats that make them pre-diabetic, overweight, and prone to heart disease later in life. In fact, the most perverted part of the Western diet is that "children's food" is high in sugar, starch, and processed fats. Think sugary cereal, processed meats, fried everything, cheese on everything, sugar-soaked everything. WHAT?!

Want to know the worst possible "food" for any human to eat—let alone humans who need the most nutrition? Look at a "kid's menu." SANE eating is a better, easier, inexpensive, and delicious way to supply children with all the calories they need.

Give children stable energy and the ability to focus and behave naturally. Starches and sweets are dramatically more Aggressive than SANE foods. They release a short burst of energy into the body. This causes a brief energy high followed by longer-lasting lethargy. Still developing mentally and emotionally, children are doubly affected by these highs and lows; that is why they start bouncing off the walls and have a hard time concentrating after eating starches and sweets. Giving a child a soda and asking them to then "behave" is like someone giving you a line of cocaine and then asking you to "behave."

SANE eating—which naturally reduces sugar and starch consumption—can go a long way toward supporting a child's overall body and brain health. It has even been "prescribed" to help kids with ADHD (attention deficit hyperactivity disorder) because it ensures a slow and steady release of energy, increases the nutritional quality of the diet, and enables optimal mood and behavior.

Set them up for success now and later. Warning: These are going to be a tough couple of paragraphs, but you've been lied to long enough, so here's two scientifically proven truths that may forever change the way you look at the way kids eat:

1. Fat cells that develop during childhood *never go away.* They can shrink, but they *forever* predispose that person to obesity.
2. Being overweight causes children more psychological trauma (think bullying, not being asked to prom, etc.) than just about any other condition.

I could rant about this for hours—and I have at SANESolution.com—but consider only this: Why are we so rightly vigilant about protecting children from smoking and secondhand smoke? Because we know it causes permanent health damage. Now consider the two *facts* about childhood obesity we just covered. Being overweight as a child causes permanent health damage AND permanent psychological damage. So why is it not only okay, but also encouraged, that our schools serve our children processed sweets, starches, and fats? Can you imagine if there was a cigarette vending machine in a grade school?

Please join me in helping our country and world see that *encouraging* our children to put things into their body that permanently harms them physically and emotionally is tragic. It won't be easy, and we won't be able to turn the tide against childhood obesity overnight, but together, we can reverse the fact that today's children are the first generation in recent history to have a lower life expectancy than their parents. We can do better. And now, armed with the facts, I'm confident we will.

Can I Cheat?

If you choose to eat something inSANE, you aren't "bad" or "off the team." If you choose to eat something inSANE, it doesn't mean you are cheating either. By the end of this book you will be able to choose how low or high you'd like your setpoint to be. SANE is not about all-or-nothing or about being perfect. The more SANE food you choose to eat, the lower your setpoint and the more you will crave SANE foods. The more inSANE food you choose to eat, the higher your setpoint and the more you will crave inSANE foods. My whole team and I are here to support you in making more and more SANE choices, so that enjoying a lower setpoint is not something you "try really hard" to do; it becomes a seamless piece of your life.

What you will find is that when you are living SANEly, all the chatter around cheating in the world of conventional dieting becomes mostly irrelevant. Your desire to cheat will drop, and if you do choose to eat something inSANE, it won't cause you to binge, to feel ashamed, or even to gain weight (thanks to your lower setpoint). And that's wonderful!

EATING OUT SANELY

Lowering your setpoint while eating out is easy and delicious if you keep the SANE Plate in mind. First, when ordering, think about how you'll get your non-starchy vegetables. Side salads and doubled portions of veggies are great options. Second, select grilled fish, steak, poultry, or any nutrient-dense protein. Keep in mind that there are many hidden fats such as oils, cheese, and butter. Tell your server that you can't have dairy and to use less oil. Use some wedges of lemon or lime, mustards, hot sauce, salsa, or vinegars as SANE condiments. Select a sugar-free beverage such as water, iced tea, or club soda with a squeeze of lemon or lime.

As for specific types of restaurants, here are SANE tips for ordering SANEly:

Restaurants for Breakfast

Easy. Eggs, meat, and veggies. Scramble, omelet, whatever you like. Breakfast is a breeze. A great go-to order you can find in most places is an egg white omelet filled with vegetables, meat, and ideally avocado. If they offer lean meats, you could do a whole-egg omelet as long as there's enough nutrient-dense protein in it to get you 30 grams of protein. Instead of hash browns or home fries, ask for sautéed or steamed non-starchy vegetables. Some diners serve lunch in the mornings, so if you are feeling nontraditional, you could even order a salad or a bunless burger.

Asian Restaurants

Again, easy. Meat or fish and double the stir-fried NSVs in place of rice or noodles. Select entrées made with steamed, grilled, or sautéed lean nutrient-dense proteins (e.g., fried duck is not a good choice). Enjoy sauces that aren't sweet. Simply ask, "Which of your sauces are MSG-free and gluten-free and contain the least sugar?"

If you are in the mood for sushi, sashimi or poke is a great choice, especially paired with mixed greens or seaweed salad.

Italian Restaurants

I'm going to stop saying "easy" because I hope you are starting to see that it is always easy to order non-starchy vegetables and nutrient-dense protein. In this case, replace pasta with non-starchy vegetables. Because of the epidemic rates of diabetes, many Italian restaurants even offer shredded or spiralized NSVs in place of pasta if you ask. Of course, let your server know that you don't need the bread basket.

Look for nutrient-dense proteins such as grilled chicken, fish, or steak. Pair your entrée with a dinner salad with an oil and vinegar dressing. Basically all "creamy" dressings you order out or buy at the grocery store will elevate your setpoint.

Mexican Restaurants

Ask for guacamole, pico de gallo, or salsa with a side of raw vegetables to use as "chips" for dipping. Order anything you want that isn't fried, wrapped in starch, served on top of starch, or smothered with cheese. Again, just ask for more non-starchy vegetables and nutrient-dense protein so you are too full for fillers like rice, tortillas, or corn. Beans (not refried beans) are fine occasionally. Ask that veggies be grilled dry, using water or very little oil.

Fajitas are perfect for SANE eating, since they are typically made with grilled meat, peppers, and onions. To make fajitas even SANEer, ask for lettuce to use in place of tortillas and request extra vegetables instead of rice.

Steakhouse

Load your plate with non-starchy vegetables: steamed broccoli, mashed cauliflower, green beans, and so forth. If there's a salad bar, you're in luck because you'll have a huge selection of fresh non-starchy vegetables.

Go for grilled salmon (or other fish), chicken breast, or steak as your nutrient-dense protein.

Middle Eastern/Greek

Choose kebabs or other grilled meat dishes. Instead of hummus, order baba ghanoush (eggplant dip) with veggies. Ask for extra vegetables or salad instead of rice or pita bread. If you are craving the flavors of a gyro, order one with a side salad and then put the gyro insides on your salad and discard the pita (some places will do this for you if you ask).

Buffet-Style Restaurant

Here's where it's really easy to create a SANE Plate. The beauty of buffets is that there are plenty of choices. Focus on steamed or raw non-starchy vegetables, or make a nice salad from salad-bar veggie choices, along with other delicious SANE foods such as hard-boiled eggs, olives, or avocado.

Select steamed shrimp, fish, turkey, or roast beef to round out your plate.

Deli

Great choices for your nutrient-dense proteins are sliced turkey, ham, chicken, or beef.

As for vegetables, enjoy a large portion of sauerkraut, a deli pickle, or a side salad. Some places will even wrap all the fillings for a sandwich in lettuce leaves or just put it on top of a salad instead of the bread. If you don't know, it never hurts to ask! Remember, if you order a sandwich, you don't have to eat the bread. Strip down the sandwich yourself and eat just the insides (like the lettuce tomatoes, pickles, and meat).

Fast-Food Restaurants

These are easier than you might think. Order a grilled chicken sandwich or a burger, along with a salad. Ditch the bread and put the contents of your sandwich on your salad and enjoy. Some fast-food restaurants will even do a lettuce-wrapped burger if you ask.

Other SANE choices include entrée salads such as a chef's salad or a chicken Caesar salad. See what other salads may be available on the menu, too. Make sure to skip the dressings, though, as those found at most fast-food restaurants are like kryptonite for your setpoint.

Many fast-food restaurants offer entrées such as baked fish or roasted chicken. Pair those with steamed veggies or a side salad.

Entertainment/Sport Events

These venues are a little more challenging but still doable. Focus on choices such as turkey legs, all-beef hot dogs without the bun, a small pack of almonds or other nuts, and large dill pickles.

Convenience Stores

If you're on the go and need a SANE meal, you'll be surprised at what you can pick up at a convenience store: 7-Eleven, for example, has packs of hard-boiled eggs, beef jerky, almonds, low-sugar protein bars, and sometimes even cut veggies or whole oranges.

Parties

Fill up on fresh vegetables and choose any nutrient-dense protein that is available. Bring one or two of your own SANE dishes for everyone to enjoy (and they will!).

Instead of a cocktail, enjoy some club soda with a twist of lemon or lime.

SANE SOS

Honestly, you may run into situations in which there won't be SANE options. A good strategy is to bring a very low-sugar, all-natural protein bar and to have a complete SANE meal before you go out. You'll feel full, satisfied, and free to enjoy your event without stressing over food. If you arrive at an event and are blindsided by the lack of SANE options, giving yourself permission to pick up something SANE to eat after the event can make it easier to resist inSANE party foods. Keeping a SANE bar in the glove box of your car can save the day in situations like this as well.

SANE Points

1. Use the SANE Plate for meal planning, a simple, visual way to eat SANEly.

2. With its wide array of food choices and their positive effect on your setpoint and overall well-being, SANE is the new definition of healthy.

3. Enjoy delicious SANE substitutions for starches and sweets in order to increase your consumption of non-starchy vegetables and fat-burning whole-food fats.

4. SANE snacks and desserts are perfect when you need a little energy boost or are simply craving a sweet, salty, or crunchy treat.

5. SANE desserts are optional but an excellent way to provide extra nutrition.

6. SANE meals are ideal for the entire family, including kids because SANE foods supply all the nutrition and calories required for growth and development—plus prevent the emotional pain and poor health of childhood overweight and obesity.

7. As SANE eating becomes integrated into your life, "cheating" will become irrelevant.

8. You can eat SANEly at any restaurant and you likely already do sometimes. Now you'll just do it consciously by using the concept of the SANE Plate to create your meals.

CHAPTER 9

Cooking and Every Recipe You'll Ever Need

If a lower setpoint required daily grocery shopping, complex cooking every time you eat, or only shopping at farmer's markets or Whole Foods, I would have a high setpoint. None of that is required to deliciously lower your setpoint.

When you start cooking SANEly, you will spend less time cooking than you spend eating, and likely save some money, too. You're going to discover how to create thousands of recipes—without spending hours in the kitchen or a fortune on food. Think of this approach as having a recipe for recipes. If you have a recipe, you can cook one meal. If you have a recipe for recipes, you can cook every meal you'll ever want. It's easy, convenient, and a fast paint-by-numbers approach—like making smoothies and SANE Plates—that you will love.

Are you ready?

The SANE Recipe for Recipes is this simple:

> 1 nutrient-dense protein + 3 non-starchy vegetables + (optional) 1 SANE whole-food fats + 1 seasoning or SANE condiment = A delicious and complete setpoint-lowering SANE meal.

Nutrient-Dense Proteins	Non-Starchy Vegetables	Whole-Food Fats	Seasonings	SANE Condiments
Anchovies	Alfalfa	Avocado	Allspice	Capers
Bison	Alfalfa sprouts	Chia seeds	Basil	Chili sauce
Catfish	Arugula	Cocoa/cacao	Caraway	Enchilada sauce
Chicken	Artichoke	(undutched)	Cardamom	Flavor extracts
Clams	Asparagus	Cacao nibs	Celery seed	Fresh herbs
Cod	Bean sprouts	Coconut	Chili powder*	Garlic, minced
Cornish hen	Beets	Coconut flour	Cinnamon*	Horseradish
Cottage cheese, low-fat	Bell peppers	Coconut milk	Clove	Hot sauce
Crab	Bok choy	Whole Eggs	Coriander	Mustards (yellow, Dijon, and brown)
Croaker	Broccoli	Olives	Cumin	
Egg whites	Broccoflower	Nuts and seeds of choice	Curry	Nutritional yeast (makes a good substitute for cheese)
Elk	Brussels sprouts		Dill	
Flounder	Cabbage		Dry mustard powder	
Grass-fed beef	Carrots		Garam Masala	Relish, dill
Haddock	Cauliflower		Garlic powder*	Salsa
Halibut	Celery		Ginger	Shiraki sauce
Herring	Chard		Marjoram	Soy sauce/tamari
Ham	Cucumber		Mint	Spaghetti sauce
Lamb	Eggplant		Nutmeg	Steak sauce
Lean conventional beef	Endive		Onion powder*	Sun-dried tomatoes
Liver	Garlic		Oregano*	
Lobster	Greens (beet, collard, mustard, turnip, and so forth)		Paprika*	Tahini
Mackerel	Kale		Parsley*	Vinegars, all types
Mahi-mahi	Kelp		Red pepper flakes*	Worcestershire sauce
Mussels	Leeks		Rosemary*	
Octopus	Mixed greens		Sage*	
Organ meats	Mushrooms		Tarragon	
Oysters	Onion		Thyme	
Plain Greek yogurt, low-fat	Peppers (all varieties)		Turmeric*	

Nutrient-Dense Proteins	Non-Starchy Vegetables	Whole-Food Fats	Seasonings	SANE Condiments
Pollock	Romaine lettuce			
Pork	Seaweed			
Protein powders (unflavored): hemp, pea, rice, and whey protein powders	Spinach			
	Sugar snap peas			
	Summer squash (zucchini, yellow squash, crookneck, pattypan)			
Rabbit				
Salmon				
Sardines/ Anchovies	Tomatoes			
	Watercress			
Scallops				
Sea bass				
Shad				
Shrimp				
Snapper				
Sole				
Squid				
Swordfish				
Tilapia				
Tofu				
Trout				
Tuna				
Turkey				
Venison				
Whitefish				

* These are SANE go-to spices that you'll definitely want to have on hand. You can add others to your spice cabinet as your cooking needs warrant.

MATCHING SANE FOODS TO SEASONINGS

Spices and herbs take foods from disappointing to delicious. Not only that, they are excellent sources of disease-fighting antioxidants. Others have anti-inflammatory effects, promote gut-healing, or enhance insulin function—all of which help lower setpoint.

Here is a list of complementary spices and herbs that can serve as a handy resource for making a shopping list for your spice cabinet and having on hand to use in SANE cooking. Each nutrient-dense protein and non-starchy vegetable is matched up with their appropriate herbs and spices.

You can also experiment with various combinations of the complementary spices that you enjoy most to enhance the flavor of the food for which it is recommended. If you're not familiar with a spice or herb, sprinkle a bit of it into a bowl and taste it.

Nutrient-Dense Proteins	Seasonings
Beef	Basil, cayenne pepper, chili powder, cumin, curry, dry mustard powder, garlic powder, onion powder, oregano, rosemary, sage, thyme
Fish	Cayenne pepper, curry, celery seed, dill, lemon juice, marjoram, mint, dry mustard powder, onion powder, paprika, parsley, sage, tarragon, thyme, turmeric
Lamb	Basil, cinnamon, cumin, curry, garlic powder, marjoram, mint, onion powder, oregano, rosemary, sage, savory, thyme
Poultry	Basil, chili powder, cinnamon, curry, garlic powder, marjoram, mint, onion powder, paprika, parsley, rosemary, sage, tarragon, thyme
Pork	Allspice, caraway celery seed, cloves, coriander, ginger, dry mustard powder, paprika, sage
Veal	Curry, dill, ginger, lemon juice, marjoram, mint, oregano, onion powder, paprika, parsley, sage, tarragon
Eggs	Basil, curry, dry mustard powder, onion powder, paprika, parsley, tarragon.

Cooked Non-starchy Vegetables	Seasonings
Asparagus	Dill, tarragon, curry, dry mustard powder, white pepper, lemon juice
Artichoke	Parsley, oregano, thyme
Beets	Basil, tarragon, allspice, coriander, ginger
Bell peppers	Basil, oregano, parsley, rosemary, thyme, curry, ginger, nutmeg, dry mustard powder

Cooked Non-starchy Vegetables	Seasonings
Bok choy	Garlic powder, ginger, red pepper flakes
Broccoli	Dill, mint, oregano, curry, ginger
Brussels sprouts	Basil, dill, parsley, dry mustard powder, nutmeg, paprika
Cabbage	Dill, mint, thyme, coriander, ginger
Carrots	Basil, parsley, thyme, coriander, curry, ginger, nutmeg, cinnamon
Cauliflower	Basil, thyme, garlic powder, onion powder, thyme, curry, nutmeg, paprika
Chard	Marjoram, parsley, allspice, nutmeg, paprika
Celery	Basil, dill, mint, parsley, curry, paprika
Eggplant	Basil, oregano, Italian spices, rosemary, thyme, curry
Greens (beet, collard, mustard, turnip, etc.)	Garlic powder, curry, cumin, rosemary, basil
Green beans	Basil, dill, oregano, garlic powder, rosemary
Kale	Caraway, dill, marjoram, tarragon, thyme, allspice, coriander
Mushrooms	Marjoram, nutmeg, parsley, oregano, basil, garlic powder, sage, tarragon, thyme
Onions	Basil, parsley, thyme, clove, curry, paprika
Spinach	Basil, rosemary, dill, thyme, allspice, nutmeg
Summer squashes	Marjoram, parsley, onion powder, sage, thyme, allspice, curry, ginger
Tomatoes	Basil, oregano, garlic powder, onion powder, parsley, rosemary, curry, paprika
Turnips	Basil, caraway, dill, marjoram, parsley, rosemary, allspice, dry mustard powder
Zucchini	Basil, oregano, rosemary, garlic powder

Tip: Use one to three herbs or spices to a recipe to enhance the flavor.

SANE CONDIMENTS

SANE eating never has to be boring or bland. In addition to using seasonings, you can turn any food into a sensational meal with the following condiments. Some like mustard or hot sauce even help to heal your metabolism.

Stick with condiments that are all natural and low or no sugar. Spend a few extra minutes examining labels at the grocery store, and avoid any product containing any inSANE sweeteners (see list in Chapter 6) or processed oils (e.g., canola, soybean, vegetable, and safflower). If you can't find these options in your grocery store, search for them online. Simply Google "all natural no sugar condiments."

IF YOU DON'T LIKE TO COOK

The SANE Recipe for Recipes system works for everyone, but it's especially helpful if you don't like to cook or you're new to cooking. Whatever your level of experience and interest, here's how to make this system work for you:

1. Lightly coat a pot with coconut oil (less than 1 teaspoon) or add a layer of water.[8]

2. Add your raw protein and brown the protein over low-medium heat for a couple of minutes—both sides.

3. Add your veggies (frozen or fresh) and stir. It is perfectly fine to microwave, cook, sauté, roast, or grill your vegetables separately, too.

4. Cover and cook for 5 to 15 minutes over medium heat, or until done. Cook everything a little longer if you need to.

5. Add 1 or 2 spices or herbs or condiments of choice and stir.

6. Serve your dish on your SANE Plate, and enjoy. That's all there is to it.

Adding more than one ingredient from each column works deliciously, as well. The SANE Recipe for Recipes system is a simple equation. As long as you put together SANE foods you like, you've got it made. Be creative!

But before you get turned loose, let's prepare a sample SANE dish, using your

---

[8] Water is the perfect ingredient to initiate cooking. It helps lessen the formation of advanced glycation end products (AGEs) that occur during the browning process, which can cause premature aging and disease. Excess AGEs form when food is exposed to direct heat and/or high heat. Cooking on lower temperatures with water creates a buffer between the food and the heat source, so it's the SANEst cooking method (less inSANE oil required and fewer disease-causing AGEs are created). You can try my hybrid technique of using about a quarter inch of water and then cooking your meat until the water evaporates. This gives you some of the browning action but fewer of the AGEs.

best friend or your worst enemy in the kitchen: chicken breasts. They are an excellent standby nutrient-dense protein when you need to get a healthy dinner on the table fast, but their bland flavor can be boring unless you spice it up.

Coat your pot as directed above (use either a small dab of coconut oil or water). Add 4 chicken breasts in a single layer and some water; cook on medium-high heat on both sides until slightly brown, about 8 minutes each side, depending on the thickness of the breasts. Add 2 large green bell peppers, cut in ½-inch squares; 2 large onions, cut in thin wedges; 1 teaspoon minced garlic (about 1 large clove); 2½ cups chopped tomatoes; and ½ cup small pitted green olives, sliced. Cook on medium-high heat for another 10 minutes, stirring often, until veggies are soft. Check that the chicken is 165°F. Sprinkle over paprika, salt, and pepper. Stir to combine. Voila: This makes a delicious SANE meal all in one pot. (If you want to cook faster, cut the chicken breasts into chunks instead of whole breasts.)

IF YOU ENJOY COOKING

Do you love to cook? If so, you are covered as this book features 30 setpoint-lowering SANE Recipes, and there are more than 1,600 other recipes on SANESolution.com. You will find both simple and some little bit more elaborate recipes to reflect the diversity of the SANE options available to you. Either way, they are all easy to put together with no-fuss preparation.

Also, if you have your own nice library of cookbooks, simply SANEitize (see substitutions in Chapter 8) your favorite recipes, replacing inSANE ingredients with their SANE substitutes. For example, replace typical starches with non-starchy vegetables: Try grandma's spaghetti sauce over spaghetti squash instead of traditional pasta. Replace potato chunks in a stew with cauliflower or radish. Substitute Greek yogurt in place of sour cream in dips and sauces or make a cauliflower-based pizza crust, instead of a flour one. Ditch the refined flour in baked goods, and use coconut flour, almond flour, or other nut flours instead. If you have a specific flavor or dish in mind, our SANE Certified Coaches are happy to help SANEitize anything you can imagine. You can connect with them and more recipes than anyone could ever cook in a lifetime at SANESolution.com.

IF YOU'RE TOO BUSY TO COOK

Busy? Me too! Here's how to save time while lowering your setpoint:

- Buy precut vegetables, frozen vegetables, and ready-made salads at the supermarket. Stock up on other convenience items such as minced garlic.
- Try batch cooking. Every time you cook, prepare enough for two meals: one you will eat now and one you will eat later. Many people take this two steps further and create enough for four meals every time they cook: one that they enjoy immediately, another that they enjoy the next day, and two meals' worth that they freeze and enjoy the following week. By following this routine, you can significantly reduce the amount of time you spend in your kitchen.
- Make use of leftovers. Leftover veggies can give soups, smoothies, and other dishes a nutritional boost. Dice leftover cooked vegetables or proteins and add them to a salad or stew. Freeze extra servings of soups or stews and other dishes in suitable containers or single-serve bags to use later in the week for quick meals.
- Fill your freezer with veggies, prepared side dishes, and even a healthy frozen meal for those days that don't go as planned.
- Do once-a-week food prep. If you can get a week's worth of dinners prepped in an hour each week, you'll save so much time and make SANE meals work for your family. Some of our most successful members do all of their cooking on weekends and have fridges and freezers packed with SANEity to start the week.
- Rotisserie chickens are one of the best time-saving foods you can buy at the supermarket. The beauty of a precooked chicken is that it can be sliced, diced, or shredded to use in salads, lettuce wraps, stir-fries, chilis, stews, or soups. Look for other precooked foods that offer convenience, such as hams or bags of fajita chicken strips.
- When it's on sale, buy and cook a large batch of ground chicken or turkey all at once and freeze it in the portions recipes call for. Doing this will cut your cooking time in half.

- Steam your veggies fast in the microwave. Place them in a glass casserole dish with a few tablespoons of water. Cover and cook on high about 5 minutes, until tender-crisp and still bright green.
- Use a slow cooker. In the morning, toss everything in—your non-starchy veggies, nutrient-dense proteins, and seasonings. Cook on low, and by dinnertime, your meal is ready.
- For SANE vitamin water, freeze slices of lemon in ice cube trays for on-the-go lemon water. You can also try strawberries or whatever low-fructose fruit you like.
- Consider buying your groceries online (many local food retailers are offering this service) and having them delivered. The less time spent at the store, the faster your prep time and the less time spent cooking.
- Keep your pantry, fridge, and freezer well stocked with items like broth, canned tuna, condiments, vinegars, olive oil, coconut oil, herbs and spices, prewashed lettuces and other greens, shredded carrots or cabbage, frozen vegetables, chicken breasts, steaks, and much more. That way, you can whip up something fast when you don't have time to shop.
- Enlist your family's help. Meal planning, prep, and cooking can be a lot for a busy person to handle. Involve your family, especially your kids. One of the best ways to get your children to eat SANEly is to engage them in food prep and cooking. Less work for you and more time with the family is a win-win.

IF YOU NEED TO SAVE MONEY

Here's the most controversial thing I'm going to say in this book: You can eat SANEly for less money than it costs to eat inSANEly. We could spend the rest of the book on this, and you can learn lots more on SANESolution.com, but here's how to get 80 percent of the value with 20 percent of the effort:

- Buy in bulk. You can cut the cost of going SANE by more than half if you do your grocery shopping at bulk wholesalers like Costco and Sam's Club. If you do not have access to these options, you can still save at conventional grocery stores. Simply wait till nutrient-dense protein and non-starchy vegetables are on sale, and then stock up and freeze what you can't use right then. Even if you live alone, you can take advantage of buying in bulk by befriending your freezer. Nearly any kind of food—except for eggs still in their shells (take them out of their shells before you freeze them)—can be frozen. To preserve food that will stay in the freezer longer than a week or two, wrap it in airtight foil, plastic wrap, or freezer paper.

- Scour sales flyers that come in newspapers or the mail and clip coupons. Sunday inserts in local papers have anywhere from $50 to $75 worth of coupons in them. Using coupons can sometimes save you up to 15 percent on your grocery bills. (Many grocery store chains offer coupons you can download to your smartphone to be scanned at the checkout counter.)
- Look for double coupons. Some supermarkets double the value of a coupon on certain days of the week, giving you extra savings on your final bill. Call your local grocery and ask if it offers this deal.
- Know your store savings programs. For example, Walmart has its "Savings Catcher" program that gives you money back if Walmart's item costs more than at a competitor's store. Walmart pays the difference, and over time, you can save a lot of money when you use this feature.
- Join a grocery savings program. Free of charge, these programs issue rewards cards and offer cardholders discounts on groceries. Signing up is as simple as filling out an application at the checkout counter.
- Stick to a budget for weekly groceries. Buy your essentials for the week and keep within the bounds of your budget.
- Purchase store brands. These often are 15 to 20 percent less expensive than their national brand counterparts, and you may not even notice a difference in quality.
- Look for marked-down items, particularly meats that haven't yet reached their expiration dates. So when you see a steak for $6.99 a pound instead of $15.99, stock up. Meats of all varieties retain their texture well in the freezer.

- Shop at times when food tends to be discounted. Sunday morning, for example, is a good time to find price cuts at grocery stores.
- Get to know your local farmer's market. Not only are you supporting local farmers, but you are also getting things that are fresh and in season, and at prices that might be a bit cheaper than you'd find at supermarkets.
- Buy non-perishable items such as canned proteins online. Numerous websites offer excellent pricing, free shipping, and additional discounts of 10 to 20 percent. For example, you can go to SANESolution.com/Amazon to see some of the canned wild-caught seafood I get from Amazon.com for absurdly good prices. SANE Grocery Shopping is as easy as 1, 2, 3.

Doesn't get much easier than this. Ready?

1. Stay on the perimeter of the grocery store (i.e., stay out of the middle aisles).[9]
2. Circle your favorites in the list below. (Tip: You can download and print more copies at SANESolution.com.)
3. Take that list to the store and—just like you do with your plate—fill your shopping cart with so many SANE non-starchy vegetables, nutrient-dense protein, whole-food fats, and low-fructose fruits that you have no room for inSANE processed starch, sweets, and fats.

Remember that like with your meals, you already grocery shop SANEly—it's just that a bit of inSANEity sneaks into your cart as well. Simply do more of what works! Crowd the packaged, processed inSANEity out with so much of your favorite fresh and frozen SANE foods and you will be a SANE shopping and setpoint-lowering superstar. To make your next trip to the grocery store as easy and SANE as possible, you can download and print free SANE grocery lists at SANESolution.com.

---

[9] That's where you'll find setpoint-elevating inSANE processed foods—because they don't need to be refrigerated or frozen.

SANE Points

- SANE cooking doesn't require a culinary degree, or even a cookbook. It's easy, convenient, and quick.
- The SANE Recipe for Recipes system is an equation you can use to create literally thousands of dishes. It involves mixing and matching nutrient-dense proteins and non-starchy vegetables and spices and herbs to create mouthwatering SANE Plates.
- Herbs and spices enhance both flavor and health. They can be your best friends when you cook SANEly.
- If you prefer to follow recipes, enjoy the recipes in this book, or feel free to experiment and SANEitize your favorites.
- Use the customizable SANE Master Shopping List each week to help you grocery-shop SANEly.
- Save money on your grocery bills by buying in bulk, taking advantage of shoppers' deals, using leftovers wisely, and cooking in bulk and freezing meals that can be reheated later.

CHAPTER 10

Diet Pills, Bad. Nutraceuticals, Good.

As you have discovered, overweight, obesity, diabetes, and diabesity are not character flaws. Rather, they are medical issues that we must treat with the same respect and diligence we would treat other potentially life-threatening diseases like cancer. They're all characterized by an elevated setpoint weight that is caused by hormonal dysregulation ("clogs"), neurological inflammation (brain inflammation), and gut dysbiosis (digestive disfunction). The good news is that these all can be reversed through SANE eating, SANE exercising (Part 4), thinking and living (Part 5), and nutraceuticals. The higher your setpoint and the further and faster you want to lower it, the more of these SANE tools you will want to leverage and the more diligently you'll want to leverage them.

Awesome! Great refresher. What the heck are "nutraceuticals"?!

That's what we'll cover in this chapter. SANE nutraceuticals are an extra-strength nutritional therapy as well as a lifelong preventative measure. Think of them like this: If you have an infection or want to prevent one, you'd take additional precautions to stop the infection, heal scar tissue, and protect against future infection. Likewise, nutraceuticals are suggested as "extras" to help clear clogs, repair your metabolism, melt away pounds, and have you looking, feeling, and living like a new person as quickly and safely as possible.

Nutraceuticals are natural components found in foods that are concentrated down to therapeutic- and pharmaceutical-grade levels. They include amino acids, vitamins, minerals, essential fatty acids, and other nutrients. Nutraceuticals are *not* diet pills. They are not a "miracle weight-loss cure." If diet pills worked, nobody would be overweight. They are also not "my" product line that this book was written to secretly sell. All the nutrients we'll cover here can be found at any reputable health food store, on Amazon, and yes…at SANESolution.com if you are interested in my company's approach to them.

With the air cleared, let's move on to understanding that these natural therapeutic compounds are clinically proven to make your setpoint-lowering eating and exercise plan far more effective, period. Do you have to take them? No. Do you "have to" eat green vegetables? No. Will you achieve a lower setpoint faster if you leverage every natural, proven, and safe tool available to you, including green veggies and nutraceuticals? Yes.

But before we get too excited, let's make sure we're on the same page about a couple of things because I realize that anything resembling "diet pills" is often rightly met with skepticism. We're not talking about diet pills. We're talking specifically about nutraceuticals. These are natural substances that are *required* by the body to make the setpoint-lowering changes you're after. Because of this, there's no question *if* nutraceuticals work—that's like questioning *if* turning your stove up will cause water to boil faster. The question can only be *how much* will nutraceuticals help. While the latter question is impossible to answer in a book because it depends on a detailed understanding of your unique situation (our SANE Coaches can help online if you are interested), take comfort in the fact that being able to question *how much* something helps instead of *if* it will help is a large step in the right direction.

Here's one quick example of this "not *if* but *how much*" distinction:

- If part of an elevated setpoint is impaired ability to mobilize fat (which it is);
- If carnitine (a recommended SANE nutraceutical) is essential to fat mobilization (which it is);
- If carnitine levels drop with age and with yo-yo dieting (which they do);
- If taking therapeutic-grade carnitine orally helps optimize carnitine levels in the body (which it does);
- Then taking therapeutic grade carnitine *will* help you reach a lower setpoint faster.

To be very clear: If you take nutraceuticals and make no other SANE changes, you will NOT achieve a lower setpoint. They work in tandem with your personalized SANE eating, sleeping, lifestyle, and exercise plan. They do not work alone.

Think of them like a catalyst for the metabolic changes you want to create in your body. A catalyst speeds up existing changes. The key phrase there is "existing changes." If you push the "turbo boost" button on a souped-up car while it is turned off in the garage, nothing happens. However, if you *first* turn the car on, get it on the racetrack, and *then* press the turbo boost...now we're off to the races!

The reason we're spending so much time talking about this smarter approach to catalyzing long-term weight loss is that there's no shortage of worthless and even dangerous diet pills out there. Some are simply ineffective, while others have been banned by the FDA.

Generally speaking, these overly hyped products either attempt to manipulate your appetite *temporarily* through suppressants or speed up your metabolism *temporarily* through stimulants. While they may work to decrease calories in or increase calories out in the short term, the *best* outcome possible is that they fail for all the same reasons eating less and exercising more fails. They do nothing to address the underlying issue: an elevated setpoint. They are bottled yo-yo dieting. They are nonsense. And that's why your long-term health and weight depend on you having a deep understanding of this more effective and safe "leverage nutraceuticals to lower your setpoint" versus "take stimulants and appetite suppressants to yo-yo diet harder and faster" approach.

One last "disclaimer" because you've been lied to enough: In the United States, the supplement industry is almost completely unregulated. This means that anyone could put sawdust in a bottle, say that it "helps optimize blood sugar," list it on Amazon, buy advertising on Facebook and Google, and legally make money selling people sawdust with the promise of a better life. I know this sounds ridiculous, but I have watched things like this happen within the wellness industry.

So while it is a fact that nutraceuticals work, it is also a fact that anyone can sell you anything and claim it's a nutraceutical. Therefore, you must proceed with extreme caution. Not caution about nutraceuticals working—they do—but caution about whether what you're buying actually contains nutraceuticals at the purity and doses necessary for them to work.

So while lowering your setpoint with SANE foods, sleep, lifestyle, and exercise, you may want an extra boost to help your metabolism heal, unclog, and get to your ideal setpoint sooner. That's where SANE nutraceuticals come in.

SANE LIPOTROPIC NUTRACEUTICALS

An important group of SANE nutraceuticals is the lipotropics. They are a clinically proven way to help your body metabolize fat for fuel (i.e., burn fat). Here is a rundown of the most powerful lipotropic nutrients.

Inositol for Preventing Fatty Liver and PCOS

Since the 1940s, this vitamin-like nutrient has been shown to assist in fat transportation and metabolism. This finding is significant, because without lipotropics like inositol, fats can get trapped in the liver. This can lead to severe problems such as cirrhosis and poor fat metabolism.

More recently, inositol has been shown to help normalize insulin levels and stabilize weight in women with "polycystic ovary syndrome" (PCOS). This is a condition defined by a cluster of symptoms in females, including obesity, insulin resistance, menstrual disorders, and the elevation of hormones such as testosterone.

Choline to Optimize Fat-Burning

An essential B vitamin, choline plays a role in the functioning of every cell in your body. Specifically, it is a special emulsifying nutrient that helps to break down cholesterol and prevents it from sticking to artery walls. It works in partnership with inositol to help the body utilize fats.

In a 2016 study of 3,214 adults, researchers checked levels of dietary choline and betaine (see below) in obese, overweight, and normal-weight men and women (Gao et al. 2016). The obese participants had the lowest levels of choline and betaine in their bodies; the overweight group had moderately low levels; and the normal-weight group had normal levels of both nutrients. Also, the lower the levels of choline and betaine, the heavier the subjects were in weight and waist circumference. Putting these findings together, we're left with the conclusion that subpar levels of both lipotropics somehow interfere with fat-burning (especially around the belly) and the inability to maintain a lower setpoint and weight.

Betaine HCl, B12, and Biotin for Enhancing Energy, Digestion, and Blood Sugar Control

This trio of nutrients plays a vital role in converting fat to energy. A derivative of choline, betaine HCl supports a healthy gastrointestinal tract and healthy protein digestion—both important for healing gut inflammation (a factor in an elevated setpoint).

A 2014 review study published in *Amino Acids* noted that doses of betaine ranging from 500 to 9,000 milligrams in both animal and human subjects suggest that betaine supplementation could promote reduced body fat and enhance lean muscle gains (Cholewa et al. 2014).

Vitamin B12 is an energy enhancer, essential to the body's energy transfer processes. It is also helpful in preventing brain inflammation. A study from the University of Oxford found that older people with a short supply of vitamin B12 were six times more likely to show signs of brain shrinkage, which is linked to impaired brain function and Alzheimer's disease (Smith and Refsum 2009). The study didn't prove low B12 levels cause brain atrophy, but it suggests that people vulnerable to deficiency, including older people and vegans, should make it a priority to get adequate B12.

A little-known member of the B-complex family of vitamins, biotin helps regulate insulin, blood sugar, and the metabolism of fats and protein. A Yale study found that 2 milligrams daily of biotin (with the mineral chromium picolinate) helped people with diabetes better control blood sugar—and lowered their cholesterol (Singer and Geohas 2006).

Methionine for Improved Cholesterol Control

This important amino acid speeds fat and cholesterol utilization and mobilizes fat from the liver to be released and used as energy. Methionine also helps the body synthesize carnitine (a fat burner) and is necessary for the synthesis of choline, making it indirectly involved in fat-burning.

In 2013, researchers at Louisiana State University Health Sciences Center published a review in *Current Diabetes Reviews*, noting that studies of methionine have shown it to improve insulin sensitivity and prevent body weight gain (Manna et al. 2013).

L-Carnitine for Fat-Burning

This amino acid shuttles newly "freed" body fat into the energy-producing power plants in your cells, the mitochondria. With help from carnitine, these amazing organelles collect fat and incinerate it to produce energy you can feel all day long.

With carnitine, there is hope for more efficient fat-burning. For example, researchers gave carnitine (250 milligrams daily) or a placebo to women with polycystic ovary syndrome. After 12 weeks, the women who supplemented with carnitine reduced their overall weight, plus trimmed fat from their waist and hips and reduced insulin resistance, compared with the placebo group, who experienced no improvements in any of these areas (Samimi et al. 2016).

In another study, 12 slightly overweight volunteers supplemented with or without carnitine for just 10 days while following a regular diet (Wutzke and Lorenz 2004). The dose was 3 grams daily. At the end of the trial, those who took carnitine had a higher rate of fat-burning than those who did not supplement. Also, the carnitine group maintained lean muscle. This means that carnitine not only burns excess body fat, but it also preserves body-defining muscle. Not bad for a single lipotropic!

Chromium Picolinate for Reducing Insulin Resistance, Fighting Cravings, and Burning Fat

This mineral helps your body better process carbohydrates while combating insulin resistance, helping to balance hormone levels and improve blood sugar levels. It also assists the body in burning fat and fighting cravings for sugar, bread, and pasta.

In a landmark study, chromium picolinate improved the action of insulin in obese, insulin-resistant rats (Wang 2006). With help from chromium, their cells were better equipped to sense and handle high-sugar burdens. The mineral enabled the cells to break down glucose, use it for energy, and lower glucose levels in the blood.

Elsewhere, a review of studies published in the scientific literature from 1966 through 2002 concluded that a daily dose of 1,000 micrograms of chromium could significantly reduce blood sugar levels in people with type 2 diabetes (Broadhurst and Domenico 2006). The review also noted that, through its involvement with insulin function, chromium may play an indirect role in lowering blood lipids.

Over a period of 8 weeks, a placebo-controlled study was conducted in overweight and obese volunteers with atypical depression to assess the effects of chromium picolinate on carbohydrate cravings (Docherty et al. 2005). Carbohydrate cravings, weight gain, sleepiness, and fatigue are characteristic symptoms of atypical depression. There were 110 patients in the study; 70 received 600 micrograms daily of chromium picolinate, and 40 took a placebo. Researchers found that daily supplementation with chromium picolinate significantly reduced carbohydrate cravings compared with the placebo. You may want chromium picolinate if you're concerned about your blood sugar levels, since this mineral plays such a key role in glucose metabolism.

Coenzyme Q10 (CoQ10) for Heart Health, Antioxidant Protection, Blood Sugar Control, and More

Whether you're lounging around at home, taking a brisk walk, or mentally tackling a complex problem, coenzyme Q10 (CoQ10) is constantly active. It's on the job, producing the energy you need for daily life. As an antioxidant, it's also defending your body from the nasty, toxic free-radical bombardment that damages your cells and ages your mind and body.

Extensively researched for an array of health benefits, CoQ10 helps convert fats and sugar to energy in cells, while protecting the heart. In fact, it has been demonstrated scientifically to help people with weak hearts, including those with diseases such as cardiomyopathy and heart failure.

A study published in 2014 in the *Journal of Diabetes and Metabolic Disorders* was undertaken to evaluate the effects of CoQ10 supplementation on lipid profiles and blood sugar control in patients with diabetes (Zahedi 2014). Fifty patients with diabetes were randomly assigned into two groups to receive either 150 milligrams of CoQ10 or a placebo daily for 12 weeks. Before and after supplementation, fasting blood samples were collected and lipid profiles containing triglyceride, total cholesterol, low-density lipoprotein cholesterol (LDL) and high-density lipoprotein cholesterol (HDL), plus fasting plasma glucose (FPG), insulin, and hemoglobin A1C (HbA1C) were measured.

Forty patients completed the study. After the experimental period, FPG and HbA1C were significantly lower in the CoQ10 group compared to the placebo group. Although blood lipids weren't affected, the researchers noted that CoQ10 appears to be an effective way to improve blood sugar control if you have diabetes. So this supplement is definitely one to have on board if you have diabetes or diabesity.

OTHER IMPORTANT SANE NUTRACEUTICALS

EPA and DHA for Fighting Inflammation

The root of so many diseases—atherosclerosis, arthritis, cancer, dementia, digestive problems, even obesity—is inflammation, so wouldn't it be amazing if you could use something natural to reduce it?

You can. Here is where eicosapentaenoic acid (EPA) and docosahexaenoic acid (DHA) come to your rescue. Known as marine omegas because they're found primarily in seafood and seaweed, both are key building blocks for some of the body's most powerful anti-inflammatory substances.

At pharmaceutical grades and in therapeutic doses, these powerful omega-3 fats directly reverse and heal neurological inflammation, which elevates your setpoint. Please note that generic "omega-3s" do not do the same thing as these specific fats, so you must purchase supplements labeled as pharmaceutical grade, which generally means that they're ultra-purified and highly concentrated omega-3 fish oils.

Vitamin D3 for Reducing Insulin Resistance, Fighting Brain Inflammation, and Protecting the Body against Diseases

Part of the steroid hormone family, which includes cortisol, estrogen, progesterone, and testosterone, vitamin D3 is a potent and active form of vitamin D, the type naturally produced in the body when skin is exposed to sunlight. Some experts believe that many people unknowingly suffer from vitamin D deficiency. A short supply of this nutrient leads to health problems that include diabetes and obesity.

In recent years, several teams of investigators have pointed out that people who are obese (especially with fat distributed around the belly) tend to have low levels of this lifesaving vitamin. No one is exactly sure why, but there's a theory. Researchers speculate that vitamin D may become trapped inside fat tissue so that less of it is available to circulate inside the blood.

If someone is obese *and* has a vitamin D deficiency, trouble really brews. This combination increases the risk of insulin resistance more than either factor alone. That's a finding reported by a team of researchers from the Drexel University School of Public Health in the journal *Diabetes Care*, after studying vitamin D levels in obese volunteers (Kabadi et al. 2012).

Also, an analysis of 28 studies concluded that people with high blood levels of vitamin D have a low risk of developing certain diseases, including cardiovascular disease, type 2 diabetes, and metabolic syndrome, a forerunner to diabetes (Parker et al. 2009).

We can't leave a story about vitamin D3, weight, and diabetes without talking about setpoint. Here's why: An adequate, healthy supply of this nutrient helps heal neurological inflammation (a major setpoint-elevating factor). The brain relies on vitamin D for protection against a variety of destructive, inflammatory processes, many of which lead to cognitive decline, stroke, Alzheimer's disease, Parkinson's disease, and other brain conditions. Whatever your situation, it's a good idea to take vitamin D3 every day for protection and neurological healing.

Probiotic and Prebiotic Nutraceuticals for Healing Gut Inflammation

SANE emphasizes foods that heal gut inflammation and build the population of gut bacteria that is associated with a lower setpoint. Beyond food, there's even more you can do to enhance the healthy setpoint-lowering bacteria that live in your gut: supplement your diet with probiotics and prebiotics.

Probiotics supply friendly digestive bacteria, and prebiotics feed these bacteria with the right nutrients. It's worth noting here that many SANE foods are prebiotic: asparagus, onions, garlics, leeks, artichokes, SANEBars, and berries, to name a few. Taking both probiotics and prebiotics together is known as *symbiotic supplementation*, and it can have a dramatic impact on your health, weight, and setpoint. If your goal is insurance against gut problems or inflammation, taking a probiotic and a prebiotic, in addition to eating gut-health-promoting SANE foods, is a great move.

L-Leucine for Muscle Health and Fat Burning

To burn fat instead of muscle, nutrient-dense protein is essential, in part because it is high in the amino acid leucine. Among amino acids, leucine is the most powerful at stimulating muscle protein synthesis (MPS). This process describes the body's ability to synthesize protein to repair and develop calorie-hungry lean muscle tissue.

In one clinical study demonstrating leucine's power in stimulating MPS, eating more leucine enabled people to lose 7 pounds more weight, while sparing lean muscle tissue, when compared with people eating the exact amount of calories but without leucine.

And in a 2003 study at the University of Illinois at Urbana–Champaign, 24 overweight middle-age women were divided into two groups, each consuming 1,700 calories a day for 10 weeks (Layman et al. 2003). One group followed the U.S. Department of Agriculture's Food Guide Pyramid and ate 0.36 grams of protein per pound of body weight every day; the second group ate twice the protein (0.73

grams), selecting high-leucine foods. Both groups lost an average of 16 pounds, but the high-protein group lost more body fat and less muscle—exactly the results you want when lowering your setpoint and reaching your ideal weight.

Some studies suggest that when you want to lose body fat and preserve muscle, taking in 2 grams of leucine along with your complete SANE meals can be helpful. If you are using clean whey protein in your SANE Meal Smoothies, you're already supplementing with leucine. Whey protein (see below) is high in leucine.

L-Glutamine for a Healthy Gut and Lower Setpoint

Another highly beneficial amino acid is glutamine, the most abundant amino acid in the body. It is the favorite fuel for your gastrointestinal cells (they prefer it over carbs and fat) and can effectively heal the soft tissue and inflammation in your gut—key benefits in lowering your setpoint.

Oral supplementation with glutamine can also favorably alter the composition of gut bacteria. Remember, there's a link between obesity and the type of bugs in your gut. Very heavy people tend to have a significantly higher number of one of the two main types of bacteria found in the gut: Firmicutes. This seems to make them prone to gaining weight. Naturally, you want to do everything you can to create a setpoint-lowering environment in your gut, and supplementing with glutamine seems to help.

ZMA for Muscle-Preservation, Hormone Balance, and Metabolism

Zinc monomethionine aspartate/magnesium aspartate (ZMA) has become a popular supplement that combines well-absorbed forms of zinc, magnesium, and vitamin B6. Zinc is essential to muscle protein synthesis, cell division, and metabolism. And magnesium is vital to the health of your bones, nerves, and immune system.

In ZMA, the combination of nutrients supports proper hormone balance in the body. For example, ZMA naturally boosts testosterone and blunts cortisol—two actions that help the body burn fat and develop muscle more effectively. The zinc in ZMA can keep your metabolic rate up and body fat down by maintaining healthy levels of your thyroid hormone. Thyroid hormone is important for helping you burn more calories and fat throughout the day. What's more, ZMA helps keep you lean by enhancing normal leptin release from fat cells. Leptin also helps increase your metabolism and curb your hunger.

Supplementing with ZMA thus supports fat-burning, enhances muscle growth, and helps regulate hunger—all key factors in lowering your setpoint.

CLEAN WHEY PROTEIN IN SANE SMOOTHIES AND BAKED GOODS

SANE smoothies are truly the most potent, natural, therapeutic, and convenient source of setpoint-lowering nutrition in the world—especially if you power them with nutraceutical-like compounds such as cinnamon, superfood powders, guar gum, konjac root, gelatin, and the other ingredients detailed in Chapter 7.

When blending a SANE Meal Smoothie, you're adding protein to the mix, and one of your choices is clean whey protein. Before we leave this chapter, I want to cover this powerful and beneficial nutraceutical in more depth so that you understand its unique value in lowering your setpoint.

There is no doubt about it: Increased protein intake is universally recognized to help with weight loss. Study after study shows that getting the proper levels of the right protein in your diet encourages weight loss, boosts muscle, and helps develop lean muscle.

One of the best dietary proteins you can take is clean whey protein concentrate. Whey is a component of milk that is separated from milk to make cheese and other dairy products and is a superior protein powder. It has several amazing health benefits:

First, it is a powerful weight-control nutraceutical. A growing number of studies prove that getting high-quality whey concentrate in your diet is helpful in reaching your ideal weight. For instance, one study has shown that women who increased their intake of whey protein lost twice as much visceral fat (belly fat) as women who didn't add protein to their diet (Bortolotti 2011).

Another study demonstrated that whey protein triggers the release of compounds that stimulate the body's feel-full hormones (Chungchunlam et al. 2015). Similarly, Australian researchers discovered that a whey protein shake reduced ghrelin (the hormone that tells your brain that you're hungry) more than any other beverage—and kept volunteers feeling full for up to 4 hours (Bowen et al. 2011).

Second, whey protein is one of the most powerful substances to develop and preserve calorie-burning muscle. This is because it is extremely rich in branched chain amino acids (BCAAs)—leucine, isoleucine and valine. These are essential for muscle development, especially leucine. If you're not getting enough of these amino acids, it can be tougher to maintain lean muscle.

Third, whey protein boosts your defenses against illness. One main reason is because whey protein is high in glutathione, the most powerful antioxidant in the body. It is an amazing molecule that acts like fly paper to attract and rid the body of disease-causing free radicals and deadly toxins, such as mercury and other heavy metals. Increasing your glutathione levels by eating more whey protein is one of the most universally recommended steps to improve nearly every aspect of your health.

Fourth, whey protein helps heal "leaky gut syndrome," which occurs when the wall of the small intestine is damaged. When your body digests food, it ideally breaks food down into the smallest possible pieces, the original building blocks, that then get absorbed through the wall of the small intestines and into the bloodstream. When the wall is damaged, larger molecules slip through the wall. Leaking undigested food into the bloodstream sets in motion a chain of events: The immune system reacts, and the body thinks it's being attacked and expresses this in the form of rashes, diarrhea, joint pain, headaches, or even psychological problems like depression. Fortunately, whey contains a powerful gut-repair compound called *alpha-lactalbumin* that strengthens the barrier between the contents of the GI tract and the blood and contributes to digestive health.

Not all whey protein is created equal. When you purchase this nutraceutical, you want to make sure that it's "clean." This means that the whey protein:

- Is sourced from grass-fed cows that are not treated with antibiotics and hormones.
- Is a "concentrate" and not an isolate or hydro isolate. Isolates are inferior because they are devoid of nutritional cofactors, including minerals, naturally occurring vitamins, and fats, all of which are lost in processing.
- Is cold-processed to ensure that all the nutrients are preserved. (Many protein powders are manufactured using

high-temperature processing, which is cheaper for them but damages the protein structure, nutrients, and absorption ability.)

- Is free of additives, sugar, fillers, and toxic metals.

To ensure that you're getting a clean whey protein, carefully read the product's label and any other product description. If the ingredients contain anything other than "grass-fed whey protein concentrate," keep looking.

Sane Nutraceuticals at a Glance

Nutraceutical	Benefit and Function	Suggested Daily Dosage (taken with meals unless otherwise stated)
Inositol	Fat transportation, metabolism, and redistribution of fat; may help normalize insulin levels and stabilize weight in women with PCOS.	1,000 milligrams
Choline	Helps break down cholesterol and prevents it from sticking to artery walls. It works in partnership with inositol to help the body utilize fats.	1,000 milligrams
Betaine HCl, B12, and Biotin	Help enhance energy production and digestion, and control blood sugar.	Betaine HCl (100 milligrams), B12 (100 micrograms), and Biotin (450 micrograms)
Methionine	Helps regulate cholesterol.	1,000 milligrams
L-carnitine	Assists the body in burning fat for energy.	600 to 1,200 milligrams
Chromium Picolinate	Reduces insulin resistance, fights cravings for carbohydrates, and assists the body in burning fat.	200 micrograms
Coenzyme Q10 (CoQ10)	Helps protect heart health, works as an antioxidant, and assists in blood sugar control.	10 milligrams
EPA and DHA	Fight inflammation.	1 tablespoon of cod liver oil or 6 fish oil capsules per day
Vitamin D3	Helps reduce insulin resistance and brain inflammation; helps protect the body against many diseases.	5,000 IU

Nutraceutical	Benefit and Function	Suggested Daily Dosage (taken with meals unless otherwise stated)
Probiotics and prebiotics	Help heal the gut and promote the balance of healthy bacteria in the gut; assist in weight control.	As directed on the bottle
L-leucine	Promotes muscle protein synthesis and fat-burning.	2 grams per meal
L-glutamine	Promotes a healthy gut and setpoint-lowering bacteria.	5 grams daily
ZMA	Helps preserve muscle tissue, balances hormones, and supports metabolism.	3 capsules daily (men) or 2 capsules daily (women), preferably on an empty stomach, 30–60 minutes before bedtime
Clean whey protein	Helps control hunger hormones and weight; promotes muscle protein synthesis; enhances immunity; helps heal leaky gut syndrome.	At least 1 scoop daily in a SANE smoothie

YOUR PERSONAL NUTRACEUTICAL PROGRAM

If you are feeling a little overwhelmed, let me give you a couple of scenarios to help you get started incorporating SANE nutraceuticals simply.

If you want faster setpoint-lowering results: Consider taking lipotropics, especially inositol, choline, methionine, betaine HCL, and carnitine. Probiotics, prebiotics, and clean whey protein also have a direct impact on setpoint-lowering and are worth considering. These nutraceuticals can form a good foundational program for you.

If you're concerned about blood sugar control, consider taking chromium picolinate, vitamin D3, leucine, and glutamine—all of which play a role in insulin function and blood sugar control. If you want heart health protection, coenzyme Q10 can be helpful.

After you get started on SANE activity (see Chapters 12 and 13), clean whey protein, leucine, glutamine, and ZMA are worthwhile additions.

If you don't like fish: Be sure to add EPA and DHA to your nutraceutical program.

As you begin the 21-Day Plan, your body will go through some amazingly positive changes. Nutraceuticals will bolster those changes. Think of them as your support team for living well and becoming that naturally thin person you're destined to be.

SANE Points

- SANE nutraceuticals can help your setpoint-lowering efforts, particularly if your metabolism is very clogged due to years of yo-yo dieting.
- SANE lipotropics help your body unlock fat stores and burn fat for energy.
- Other SANE nutraceuticals help insulin function normally, improve immunity, curb cravings, heal gut inflammation, improve the population of fat-fighting bacteria, and enhance overall health.
- Like every tool available to you in building a SANE lifestyle, nutraceuticals are not required, but they will help you repair your metabolism and lower your setpoint faster if you leverage them along with every other tool in your setpoint-lowering SANE toolbox.

PART 4

SANE EXERCISE

CHAPTER 11

Exercise Less, Lower Your Setpoint More

You've been told "do more exercise." That's about as helpful as being told "take more pills." Which? When? Why? How much? For how long?

In order to achieve your health goals, first YOU must identify your specific goal, and only then can you specify which form of treatment is most appropriate. For example, imagine you went to see your doctor with the specific goal of healing your broken arm, and your doctor prescribed you cough medicine. That would be an inappropriate treatment for your desired outcome.

Type of Treatment	Goal
Cast	Repair a broken bone
Cough syrup	Reduce coughing
Metformin	Manage diabetes
Zoloft	Manage depression
Ibuprofen	Reduce inflammation
Cardiovascular exercise	Manage depression
SANE activity	Lower setpoint
Stretching	Relieve muscle cramps
Trendy workout DVDs	Make celebrity richer

If you want to run a marathon, there's a specific form of exercise that will help you do that. If you want strong biceps, there is a specific form of exercise that will help you do that. And if you want *lasting* weight loss, there is a specific form of exercise that will lower your setpoint—which is the *only* way to do that.

Assuming that you are not already a SANE member, you likely have never done the specific forms of exercise that lower your setpoint. If you have exercised in the past, or are exercising now, perhaps you've aimed for other goals, such as strength, cardiovascular fitness, flexibility, and so forth. That's fantastic, and those are great goals, but this isn't a program about those goals; it's specifically designed to do one thing, and one thing only: lower your setpoint so that you can become naturally thin for life. That's it.

If you have turned to this chapter, thinking it will be page after page of how to exercise more to lose weight, don't worry. It is none of that. You are going to learn about a revolutionary form of physical activity that you can begin no matter what your current fitness level is, at home, with no expensive equipment.

WHY EATING LESS AND EXERCISING MORE DOESN'T WORK

Forget everything you've ever heard about exercise. Forget about "target zone," "go for the burn," "take it to the max." Forget about exercising more to lose weight. For lowering your setpoint, none of this works—and that's according to *Journal of the American Medical Association* (Ludwig and Friedman 2014) and many other scientific studies.

In the same way that you are focusing on the *quality* of what you eat instead of counting calories (*quantity*), you can lower your setpoint by focusing on the *quality* of your activity—and not the calories burned (*quantity*) or the time you spend working out (*quantity*). Simply looking at calories burned is harmful because it ignores how exercising more can hurt your hormones, metabolism, and setpoint— and ultimately your ability to stay naturally thin.

It's time to talk about a new way to move your body—one that ignores calories in the short term and instead focuses on lowering your setpoint long-term: SANE activity. There are three forms of SANE activity, which I'll cover in this chapter and the next: "eccentric" training, a type of movement that accentuates the lowering part of a movement; smarter interval training, which involves short, intense, but *safe* bursts of work followed by periods of lower-intensity work; and restorative activity, which can be anything from yoga to a nature walk and is designed to reduce setpoint-elevating stress hormones.

"Exercise more" is simply an unhelpful recommendation. What does this even mean? What is exercise? If you talk to a weight lifter, she might define exercise differently than your walking buddy, who might define it differently than an Olympic swimmer, who might define it differently than the mom down the street with five kids.

And how long is "more"? More than what? If you exercise more today than you did yesterday, does that mean tomorrow you have to exercise even more? And what about the day after? And the day after that? This is just as absurd as the advice to just eat less.

In fact, the theory that we have an obesity epidemic because people are not exercising enough is disproved by other data. In a July 2013 report, the *Institute for Health Metrics and Evaluation* found that "as physical activity increased between 2001 and 2009, so did the percentage of the population considered obese" (Murray et al. 2013).

Because typical exercise advice focuses on burning calories, exercisers spend their time in the gym, staring at the calorie estimator on a piece of aerobic equipment ticking away. Not only are those calorie estimators wildly deceptive and as inaccurate as the nutrition labels on packaged foods, but they are also the exact wrong issue to focus on. Instead of worrying about the *quantity* of exercise, the focus needs to be on the *quality* of exercise. Fortunately, scientific research has demonstrated that if you pursue the high-quality movements you'll learn here, the results are therapeutic to your setpoint, metabolism, and overall health.

Case in point: A study done at Skidmore College compared a traditional calorie-counting "eat less, exercise more—harder" program against a simpler "eat more, exercise less" program (Arciero et al. 2006).

There were two groups in this study. Let's call them the Quantity Group and the Quality Group. The Quantity Group ate a more conventional Western diet, while performing traditional aerobic exercise for 40 minutes per day, 6 days per week. The Quality Group followed a smarter diet, while exercising only 60 percent as much, but with higher quality. The study lasted 12 weeks and included 34 women and 29 men between the ages of 20 and 60.

At the end of the study, the Quantity Group ate less food and exercised 18 hours more than the Quality Group. The Quality Group focused on high-intensity cardio and resistance training and ate more but higher-quality calories. Here's what the researchers found:

Quality Group vs. Quantity Group

The Quality Group lost more body fat, developed more body-firming muscle, trimmed their waistlines significantly, and dropped their cholesterol levels. Amazing, isn't it?

What this means to you: The movement principles you will learn and apply here will have the same transformative effects on you because they will lower your setpoint.

If you are thinking, "But I like to jog" or "I enjoy going to my Zumba class," that's fine, and you should continue doing what you enjoy. If you love going to a Zumba class, dancing, and being with your friends, that is wonderful. Those specific types of exercises are great at some things. They're just not great at the specific type of setpoint-lowering effects we're after here. SANE activity is the form of exercise that lowers your setpoint most effectively. Best of all, you can do very little of it, infrequently, and sit back and enjoy those results.

And for what it's worth, it's rare in life that you can do less and get more. So when that opportunity arises—like it is right now—enjoy it!

HORMONES, SETPOINT, AND SANE ACTIVITY...OH MY!

This new way of moving your body activates positive hormonal changes, which lower your setpoint. Traditional exercise such as aerobics, extreme aerobics, jogging, and running activate negative hormonal changes that can raise your setpoint.

For example, traditional exercise suppresses the production of the thyroid hormone T3 (a key hormone in determining if your body can "burn more"—instead of store more—when faced with excess calories), especially in women. The last thing you want is for exercise to harm T3 production, slow down your metabolism, and cause your body to store more fat.

Also, traditional exercise can exert a lot of stress on your body. The American Heart Association found that jogging injures more than half of the people who do it. This high injury rate is due in part to the fact that every mile you run, your feet hit the ground about 900 times. Let's say you weigh 150 pounds. That means for every mile you run, you are smashing 135,000 pounds of force against your joints, ligaments, and every other part of your body. You could say that's like dropping 37 Toyota Camrys on yourself every time you go for a jog.

Even worse is the hormonal damage involving cortisol. I know we already talked about cortisol quite a bit, but because of all that "exercise is so amazing and healthy for you" messaging out there, it's critical to understand that exercise raises your stress, or cortisol, levels. As you learned in previous chapters, chronic high levels of this hormone *cause* a high setpoint. Few things are this clear in human metabolism, but the fact is that studies always show that if you chronically elevate cortisol (like when you go to bed late every day because of work and then force yourself to get up early to exercise), your setpoint will rise. You may also remember that elevated cortisol is particularly detrimental to your waistline, as it causes a disproportionate amount of fat to deposit around your midsection.

To add insult to injury, chronic stress also increases insulin levels. As you now know, chronically high insulin, like cortisol, directly *causes* a high setpoint in humans. In human study after human study, if you elevate humans' levels of insulin (e.g., through medication), their setpoint rises. It's a setpoint double whammy when you are chronically stressed out!

Finally, there is the negative impact that traditional exercise has on your appetite hormones—leptin and ghrelin. Research suggests that exercises such as spinning, swimming, and running increase appetite shortly after exercise by decreasing leptin and raising ghrelin. This can lead to cravings for the inSANE foods that elevate your setpoint.

When you think about the traditional forms of exercise that have failed you in the past, it's helpful to think about their impact on appetite like this: In the same way that people drink more water when they do more traditional exercise, they also eat more when they do more traditional exercise. Jeffrey M. Friedman, MD, PhD, head of the Laboratory of Molecular Genetics at Rockefeller University in New York, puts it well: "Exercise by itself has not been shown to be highly effective in treating obesity because the increased energy use from exercise is generally offset by increased caloric intake."

By contrast, SANE activity has no negative impact on appetite and powerfully helps to clear hormonal "clogs." It has been shown to reduce insulin resistance and raise levels of two fat-burning hormones—testosterone and human growth hormone (HGH)—which are essential for reducing body fat, especially belly fat. A study from East Carolina University published in 2007 in the *Journal of Applied Physiology* showed how smarter exercisers burned belly fat both during and after a workout (Hortobágyi et al. 1993 and Ormsbee et al. 2002). The researchers inserted probes in the exerciser's fat tissue. The probes stayed in place before, during, and 45 minutes after a resistance training workout (resistance training is a key part of the SANE plan). At the end of the workout, researchers found that resistance training increased the burning of belly fat during exercise and for at least 40 minutes afterward.

If you are serious about lowering your setpoint weight permanently, then incorporating SANE activity into your life should take priority over any other type of movement. Whether you are starting from active, sedentary, or somewhere in the middle, with just 20 minutes a week, you will clear away the hormonal clog that has been keeping your setpoint elevated.

INSANE EXTREME EXERCISE VERSUS SANE ACTIVITY

There has been a surge of "extreme" forms of exercise hitting the market recently. Why? This is just another iteration of the common "more is more" myth. If walking is so good for you, jogging must be twice as good. Then running a mile. But let's take that up a notch with a 5K, then a 10K, then a half marathon, then a marathon, and then an ultramarathon. More is not more, especially when it comes to exercise. Just about every orthopedic surgeon and chiropractor tells me: "CrossFit and those 'extreme' DVD workouts are the greatest thing that's ever happened to my business!" because of the injuries they almost always cause.

It can be helpful to think of these forms of physical activity like cutting your hair with a chainsaw. It may sort of "work" in some perverted sense of the word, but it also carries along with it excessive and unnecessary risk. Also, if these exercises were as potent as claimed, why would anyone need to do them 5 or more days per week? Think about the potency of exercise as being like the potency of cayenne pepper in a recipe—a little bit adds a lot of spiciness. You do not need a large quantity of potent things—and if you need a lot of something, it is not potent.

To be fair, quite a few people, from competitive endurance athletes to high-performing military personnel, swear by extreme-exercise regimens. If you enjoy extreme exercise and can do it safely and sustainably, then enjoy it. It simply doesn't lower your setpoint.

None of what I'm saying means you should ever give up on exercise. It simply means you will reach your goal faster if you exercise in a way specifically designed to get you to your specific goal.

HOW SANE ACTIVITY HELPS LOWER YOUR SETPOINT

SANE activity has nothing to do with the quantity of calories burned during the 1 percent of your life you will spend exercising. It focuses on the *quality* of how you exercise, which is to say what muscle fibers you engage, how many you activate, and how they trigger more clog-clearing hormones—thereby lowering your setpoint.

Six SANE principles come into play when lowering your setpoint through activity. Once you understand these principles, you'll see why SANE activity allows you to work out smarter, in less time, and get even better results, using a simple set of movements you can perform in just 20 minutes a week.

Principle #1: Deep

A little SANE exercise does something any amount of traditional exercise *can't* do: It stimulates your *deep* muscle fibers. For background, we all have several different types of muscle fibers that do different things. Broadly speaking, each of your skeletal muscles contain slow-twitch and fast-twitch fibers. Type 1 fibers, or slow-twitch fibers, are involved mostly in exercises that require a little force for a long time such as running, jogging, or cycling.

Fast-twitch fibers, on the other hand, are used when you need a lot of force for a short period of time, like when you are lifting a heavy piece of furniture. Fast-twitch fibers are further divided into type 2a, type 2x, and type 2b fibers—each getting progressively stronger and more hormonally helpful. These fibers are what I refer to as "deep." When you do SANE workouts, you will use type 1 and all type 2 muscle fibers, whereas traditional exercises such as jogging or running use only type 1 fibers.

Stop and think about that for a moment. You are about to do a form of physical movement that activates muscle fibers that you may have *never* activated before. How exciting is this?! Think about if you never exercised your biceps for your whole life and then started exercising them. Could you imagine how quickly you would experience dramatic results? That's a lot what you have available for you for every muscle on your body with this new method of movement. Entire classes of muscle fibers (type 2a, type 2x, and type 2b) found in every one of your skeletal muscles will be activated for the first time in your life!

Type 2b muscle fibers are especially exciting. They have the ability to lower your setpoint quickly because, when activated, they trigger a huge amount of clog-clearing hormones. Boston University researchers found that the type 2b muscle fibers have "a previously unappreciated role in regulating whole-body metabolism [unclogging]." And a big reason conventional exercise hasn't helped you *keep* weight off is because it *never* activates these types of muscle fibers (more on this below).

While working out smarter, you'll be doing slow and safe movements that require a lot of force, activate your deep muscle fibers, and demand a lot of energy. You'll then run out of energy in a short time, but you'll achieve dramatic hormonal benefits. You'll also get quite sore and won't be able to do it for a long time or frequently. And that's great: You get more results in less time.

By working your deep muscle fibers, you can work out less—but smarter—and create an incredible setpoint-lowering response that is not possible with traditional forms of exercise.

Principle #2: Resistance

To unlock the hormonally healing power of all those previously untapped muscle fibers, you must exercise with enough "resistance." Resistance training is any form of exercise that requires your skeletal muscles to contract against an opposite force (the resistance). What can you use for that external resistance? Anything you want: dumbbells, barbells, kettlebells, resistance bands, a weight vest, soup cans, bottles of water, bricks, another person, even your own body weight.

When the resistance becomes too great for your slow-twitch fibers, then your deeper fast-twitch muscle fibers are recruited. Therefore, applying enough resistance is necessary for activating your uniquely beneficial fast-twitch fibers. The more resistance you apply to your muscles (up to a point), the better setpoint-lowering results you get. It's also important to note that no quantity of light resistance will ever activate these specific setpoint-lowering muscle fibers. However, one forceful push gets the job done. That's why a lot of resistance is essential to activating your unique setpoint-lowering type 2 muscle fibers.

Because you will be incorporating a lot of resistance to ensure your muscles have to generate a lot of force, your SANE workouts will use up a lot of energy quickly and will therefore be short.[10] Also, because they are activating *all* your muscle fibers (not just your type 1 slow-twitch muscle fibers), your SANE workouts require a lot of recovery time. In fact, how long your muscles take to recover is a great way to tell if you are working out smarter. If you exercise on Monday and then can do the same workout (same reps, same weight, etc.) a day or two later, you are not activating your deep muscle fibers. But if Monday's workout used enough resistance to exercise all your muscle fibers, they will not be ready to go again 1, 2, 3, 4, or even 5 days later. Type 2b muscle fibers need *at least* 6 days to recover.

If you are exercising frequently, either you are not exercising smarter or you are not giving your deep muscle fibers enough time to do their hormonally healing job. Either way, you are spending more time exercising and burning less body fat, long-term. Enough of that. Enjoy SANE activity to do less and get more.

---

[10] Exercising with more resistance doesn't mean that you have to put more stress on your joints. The techniques that follow let you increase resistance and maximize the results of your workout without increasing the impact on your body. SANE moves are so safe that they are commonly used for physical therapy after surgery or for injuries caused by conventional high-impact or extreme forms of exercise.

Principle #3: Eccentric

Traditional resistance training exercise has two types of contraction: concentric, which occurs as the muscle is shortening, usually as you lift the resistance (e.g., curling a dumbbell up with your arms), and eccentric, which occurs as the muscle is lengthening, usually as you lower the resistance (e.g., lowering the dumbbell with your arms).

Lifting weights—the concentric action—gets more attention in muscle magazines but lowering weights—the eccentric action—gets more results in studies. In fact, safely and slowly lowering resistance enables you to use up to 40 percent more resistance. More resistance means more total muscle fibers activated, more setpoint-lowering hormones triggered, and more calorie-hungry muscle developed.

Wait! Does that mean exercising like this will make me grow big bulky muscles? Nope. Few people can become very muscular because few people—particularly women—have the genes required to do so. As William Kraemer, PhD, the editor of the *Journal of Strength and Conditioning Research*, tells us, "Women have been sold a myth of becoming big. They do not have the genetics."

There are hormonal issues at play, too. The high levels of testosterone needed to develop bulky muscles are found in only a small percentage of men, and as mentioned earlier most women have about the same level of testosterone as a ten-year-old boy. Also, everyone has a gene called *GDF-8*, which regulates a substance called *myostatin*. This controls the amount of muscle you have and how much it develops naturally. It is why some people have more natural muscle tone than others, even without exercise—they have higher levels of myostatin. The base levels of hormones, myostatin, and muscle in nearly all women and most men make it impossible for them to naturally build "bulky" muscles using any form of exercise.

Principle #4: Hormonal

Yasuhiro Izumiya, MD, PhD, a molecular cardiologist at Boston University, found that the development of the specific type of muscle fibers targeted by SANE movement "can regress obesity and resolve metabolic disorders in obese mice" (Izumiya 2008). Notably, Izumiya doesn't mention "burning calories" or "working up a sweat," but rather mentions "resolving metabolic disorders"—that is, clearing hormonal clogs.

Izumiya went on to describe how these muscle fibers cleared hormonal clogs by improving "insulin sensitivity and [causing] reductions in blood glucose, insulin, and leptin levels." Most encouragingly, he noted, "These effects occurred despite a *reduction* in physical activity." This is more proof that less is more when you want to clear hormonal clogs and lower your setpoint.

The effect on other hormones is equally profound. Exercise scientists from East Carolina University in Greenville, North Carolina, and Pennsylvania State University in University Park examined the effects of both concentric and eccentric muscle contractions on several anabolic (setpoint-lowering) hormones. The 21 test subjects were young men randomly assigned to one of three groups: an eccentric-training group, a concentric-training group, and a nonexercising control group.

The eccentric group showed increased levels of both growth hormone and testosterone—both of which favor muscle-toning and development, plus decreased secretion of cortisol (which suppresses muscle development and stores fat). These findings suggest that eccentric muscle contractions are most effective for eliciting an increased flow of anabolic hormones conducive to developing your calorie-hungry and setpoint-lowering lean muscles—and dampening the effects of fat-storing cortisol.

Eccentric exercise also helps clear up another hormonal condition: insulin resistance. A study in *Medicine & Science in Sports & Exercise* found that just half an hour of eccentric exercise a week reduced insulin resistance more than concentric exercise did (Irving et al. 2008). Twenty women were randomly assigned to an exercise group that did either concentric or eccentric movements once a week for 8 weeks. At the end of the experiment, researchers discovered that the eccentric exercisers had substantially increased muscle strength, decreased insulin resistance, and improved blood lipid profiles more than concentric exercise.

Principle #5: Infrequent

Infrequent SANE workouts can deliver lifesaving benefits without requiring hours each week. The more resistance you use and the more you accentuate the eccentric portion of the movement, the more muscle fibers you work, the more energy you use, and the more sore you get—therefore, the less exercise you need to do in terms of both duration (exercise for about 10 minutes at a time) and frequency (once or twice per week) to burn fat and lower your setpoint.

Besides the "more time to do everything else" benefits, infrequent exercising also helps keeps stress levels *down* and cortisol, that same stress hormone we've discussed a bunch, in check. Infrequent workouts also ensure your body can actually benefit from your workout. Not many people talk about this, because there's no money to be made by telling people *not* to work out, but most of the benefits from effective forms of exercise happen while you are recovering—not while you are exercising.

When you exercise effectively, you cause slight and useful damage to your body. Your body then repairs this damage and gets a little more robust to "protect" itself from future damage. If you exercise too frequently, that robustification—that is, the whole point of effective exercise—doesn't happen. Again, more is not more. Less is more. And that's why your smarter approach to exercise is all about safe, short, and infrequent workouts.

Principle #6: Brief

When you exercise all your muscle fibers, you use up all your energy quickly and therefore can't do it for a long period of time. Putting it another way, if you can do any sort of movement for a long period of time, it's not activating all your muscle fibers; it's only activating your "slow to run out of energy" slow-twitch fibers. For example, you can't hold a heavy box of books (lots of resistance/weight and a lot of muscle fibers worked) as long as you can hold this book (little resistance/weight and few fibers worked). Like the infrequency principle, this principle is awesome because it means you get radically better results from exercise and have plenty of time for all the beautiful things that your new, lower-setpoint life will have in store for you.

With brief workouts, you become completely exhausted in only a matter of seconds. That's intense. But you do this by moving in an extremely slow and controlled manner using larger muscle groups and more muscle fibers. That's safe. You put zero impact on your joints, so there's less chance of injury. That's sustainable. You will feel sore for several days after a single short workout. That's effective. In short: SANE activity actually does what "extreme" forms of exercise claim to do, but it does so in less time with dramatically more safety, sustainability, and effectiveness.

SANE INTERVAL TRAINING

The best way to exercise SANEly is by doing the eccentric training that we just covered (we'll cover the "how to" in the next chapter). However, if you enjoy using cardio machines such as stationary bikes or ellipticals to exercise, you can do those SANEly—using more resistance—too. This is called SANE interval training.

SANE interval training is like a metabolic plunger for hormonal clogs. Experts at Pennington Biomedical Research Center, for example, have found that it stimulates the body to improve insulin sensitivity more than low-quality/high-quantity cardiovascular exercise (Earnest 2008). You can also stimulate many deep muscle fibers with SANE interval training, which leads to a lower setpoint. Best of all: It takes 10 minutes a week. Again, it's awesome, and all sorts of studies prove it.

Brian Irving, PhD, of the University of Virginia, took two groups of women and had them do traditional cardiovascular exercise or SANE-type interval training (Irving et al. 2008). The two groups burned the same number of calories exercising, but the SANE-exercise group spent significantly less time exercising, while losing significantly more belly fat.

Martin Gibala, PhD, of McMaster University, separated people into SANE-type interval training and traditional cardiovascular exercise groups. Over the course of the 2-week study, the SANE group exercised for 2.5 hours, while the traditional exercise group exercised for 10.5 hours (McGuff and Little 2009).

At the end of the study, both groups got the same results even though the SANE-exercise group spent 320 percent less time exercising than the traditional exercise group. Gibala put it like this: "We thought there would be benefits, but we did not expect them to be this obvious. It shows how effective short intense exercise can be."

RESTORATIVE ACTIVITIES

The third and final form of SANE movement is restorative activities. Be sure to enjoy as much restorative activity as you can to complement your SANE eccentric and interval training. Restorative activity includes walking, recreational bike riding, yoga, Pilates, stretching, tai chi, meditation, and qigong. If you choose to include walking—which is about the easiest restorative activity you can do—10,000 steps daily is a great idea.

These activities link the body and mind through conscious movement that helps decrease the nervous system's perception of stress. This drops levels of the stress hormone cortisol, which, as you know, causes all sorts of setpoint chaos. So the takeaway is simple: Do about 20 minutes of SANE eccentric and smarter interval training per week and then focus on lots of easy and enjoyable restorative activities.

Phew! That was a lot and a lot different from what you've been told in the past. And thank goodness, because if you're like most people, conventional high-quantity/low-quality exercise hasn't left you slimmer. Instead, it's left you bored, injured, discouraged, hungrier, and heavier. Not because you did anything wrong but because the advice you were given is wrong.

Thankfully, your new smarter approach is to think of exercise like medicine and to celebrate because you just discovered the prescription for *permanent* weight loss when used in conjunction with SANE eating: 20 minutes weekly of eccentric resistance training and SANE interval training, complemented with enjoyable restorative activity. Less time spent exercising, more time spent enjoying your new lower-setpoint life. Love it!

SANE Points

- The sole purpose of SANE activity it to lower your setpoint. You can clear hormonal clogs and lower your setpoint in only 20 minutes of SANE activity a week.
- There are three forms of SANE activity: eccentric training, interval training, and restorative activity.
- Traditional forms of exercise done to extremes can be injurious and hard on your body, triggering stress and poor hormonal responses that interfere with your ability to burn fat, lower your setpoint, and control your weight.
- SANE exercises work deeply, stimulating all muscle fibers, including type 2b, which has the profound ability to lower your setpoint when activated. SANE exercise emphasizes the eccentric, or lowering, portion of resistance training. Increasing resistance and accentuating the eccentric is the only way to activate your dormant and setpoint-lowering type 2b muscle fibers.
- SANE workouts are brief and infrequent—shown in research to be more effective than long hours spent exercising.
- SANE interval training, which requires only 10 minutes a week, translates into increased fat loss, cardiovascular fitness, and a lower setpoint.

CHAPTER 12

The 20-Minute-per-Week SANE Exercise Program

The SANE exercise program takes at most 20 minutes per week, requires no expensive equipment or exercise experience, can be done at home, and can be adapted for people with special needs. In other words, the SANE exercise program will work for you! All it involves is four eccentric exercises performed for 10 minutes, once a week, along with 10 minutes of smarter interval training once a week (this can be done at home or at a gym).

Starting a new exercise program is exciting. You are looking forward to getting stronger, having more energy, looking better, and getting healthier. However, getting started can be a little overwhelming. Where do you even begin?

We can discover your perfect starting point with a simple self-test to assess your current fitness level. So let's get started right now with the simple SANE self-test below.

SANE Activity Self-Test

Read through the SANE eccentric resistance exercises below. Select one for your legs, chest, shoulders, and back—a total of four moves.

Perform half of the eccentric movement and then hold. If you can hold longer than 10 seconds at the halfway point, you need more resistance (which may involve adding dumbbells, resistance bands, or other loads to the exercise). If you cannot hold statically at all, you need less resistance.

It takes trial and error to find the appropriate resistance to start with, and I know this can be frustrating. But if you perform this self-test, you will get a better handle on how much resistance to use. It's always better to start off lighter than heavier, especially if you have been sedentary for a while, when learning how to train eccentrically. But as you progress, your body will quickly create adaptations and activate more muscle fibers.

Proper exercise form is essential to ensuring that you properly activate all your muscle fibers and avoid injury. By practicing these movements for your first couple weeks of the 21-day program, the movements will "pattern" in to your central nervous system, and proper form will become second nature to you. This frees you up to focus on moving more resistance (versus worrying if you are moving correctly), which means more muscle activation, which means better setpoint-lowering results.

SANE WORKOUT INSTRUCTIONS

Each of the following exercises can be done in the comfort and convenience of your own home. The only equipment required is a set of resistance bands, which are used on a few of these moves. Bands are an easy way to add and increase resistance. It's a good idea to purchase a set of bands that is color-coded by level of resistance. You can find these at any sporting goods store or at Walmart, Amazon, and so on.

You can increase resistance by decreasing the length of the band between your hands or by doubling up and using two bands. As you get stronger and the moves become easier to do, switch to a band with greater tension. For an additional source of resistance, you may want to invest in some dumbbells or barbells.

As you did in the self-test, select one exercise per body part—legs, back, chest, and shoulders—that fits your current fitness level for a total of four exercises. As a general guideline, repeat the move until it is impossible to lower the resistance for 10 seconds. If this takes more than 6 repetitions, gradually add resistance until it takes only 6 repetitions. The ideal eccentric workout is 1 movement per muscle group (legs, back, chest/arms, shoulder/arms, in that order of priority), 6 repetitions of 10 seconds each. If you are doing exercises using one arm or one leg at a time, do 6 repetitions of 10 seconds per limb.

For videos demonstrating all of this and more, for more information on how to work out eccentrically on gym equipment, or for info on how to exercise eccentrically given specific physical limitations, we're happy to help at SANESolution.com.

Legs
GYM EQUIVALENTS: SMITH MACHINE SQUAT, SLED LEG PRESS, SLED HACK SQUAT, SQUAT RACK WITH SAFETY BARS

Two-Legged Box Squat Start Here

- Stand with your feet shoulder-width apart in front of something sturdy that you can hold on to with both hands, such as a railing or a doorknob. Your toes should be turned slightly out.
- Place a chair behind you (if you are a beginner, start with a higher seat on the chair, and then "graduate" down to lower and lower seats until your thighs are about parallel to the floor).
- Hold the support and lean back until your arms are fully extended. Stand with all your weight toward your heels. Keep your chest up and butt out.
- Bending at the hips and at the knees, sit backward and down, slowly lowering your hips toward the chair seat to the count of 10. As you lower, keep your chest up and your knees apart from each other. Try to keep your knees from going past your toes.
- Once your hips reach the seat, return to standing. It is completely okay if you need to use your arms to help you stand back up again. This is 1 repetition.
- Repeat 6 more repetitions of lowering your hips down onto the seat.

- To increase resistance: Perform the move wearing a weight vest or by shifting more weight into just one foot, or by completely lifting one foot off the floor.

ONE-LEG NEGATIVE STEP-UP (LEGS AND HIPS)

- Stand on a raised platform, such as a bench, a stair, or an aerobic step with risers. Hold on to a railing, counter, or wall for balance. Straighten your back and pull your navel in toward your spine to brace your low back. Maintain this posture throughout the exercise.
- Stand on the edge of the platform so that your right foot is firmly on the platform and your left foot is in midair.
- Bend your right knee and hip and begin to lower your left foot toward the floor to the count of 10. Keep your torso as upright as possible. When your left foot reaches the floor, that is 1 repetition.
- Repeat for 6 repetitions. Then switch to your left leg and repeat the exercise.

Caution: This exercise is suitable for beginners but can be problematic for those with balance issues.

To increase resistance: First increase the depth of the squat (raise the height of the platform), then eventually wear a weight vest or hold a weight. This is a good move to try after you have mastered the two-legged box squat.

SPLIT SQUAT

- Step your feet out about 3 to 4 feet apart. Turn your right leg out 90 degrees and your left leg deeply in—a staggered stance. It is okay if your rear/left foot's heel is not fully in contact with the ground.
- Lean slightly forward, and put as much weight on the front foot as you can. Then "squat" down by flexing the knee and hip of

your front leg to the count of 10. Let your rear leg bend until it almost makes contact with the floor. Make sure both your knees point in the same direction as your feet throughout the movement. Imagine a straight line from the crown of your head to the knee of your back leg.

- Once your rear knee is close to the floor and the front leg's thigh is parallel to the floor, you have completed the eccentric portion of the movement.
- When complete with the eccentric lowering, simply lower the rear knee to the floor or to a folded towel and then stand back up. Alternatively, you can also just step the back foot forward to exit.
- Set up in the original standing position again. Repeat 6 times. Switch to the opposite leg and continue the exercise.

To increase resistance: Gradually shift more and more weight onto the front leg. Do this by placing the rear foot on something off the ground like a stair step, stool, or low chair. Additional resistance can be added using handheld weights or a weight vest.

Caution: Some extra care should be taken when elevating the rear foot if you have balance issues, limited mobility in your ankles, or plantar fasciitis.

Chest/Shoulders/Arms

GYM EQUIVALENT: CHEST-PRESS MACHINE, SMITH MACHINE BENCH PRESS, DUMBBELL BENCH PRESS, BENCH PRESS WITH SAFETY BARS OR A SPOTTER

Wall Push-Up Start Here

- This exercise is the most basic type of push-up. After you master it, try progressing to the other push-ups described below.
- Face a wall, standing a little farther than arm's length away. Position your feet shoulder-width apart. Place your palms flat against the wall, shoulder-width apart and parallel to your chest.
- Lean forward toward the wall, while bending your elbows and lowering your upper body toward the wall in a slow, controlled

motion. Keep your feet flat on the floor and your torso stiff. If your calves or ankles feel tight, it is okay to let your heels come up off the floor.

- This is one repetition. Repeat the exercise for the required number of repetitions. To exit the posture, simply bend your knees and walk toward the wall, then set up again with your arms straight.

Caution: If you have limited wrist mobility, you can make a fist and use padding, or get handles that you can grip and keep your wrist neutral.

To increase resistance: Increase the angle by pressing against a lower support, such as a sturdy bookshelf, dresser, chair, or stair step. Advancing from the wall to things that are progressively lower increases resistance.

KNEE PUSH-UP

- After you have mastered the wall push-up, progress to trying this move.
- Kneel on hands and knees. Place a folded blanket or towel under your knees if they are tender.
- With your arms straight, place your shoulders over your wrists. Bend your elbows and lower your upper body slowly to the ground to the count of 10. This is the eccentric part of the move. If going all the way to the floor causes discomfort in your shoulders, placing a folded blanket under your chest will prevent you from going too low.
- When your nose gets close to the floor, that is 1 repetition. To set yourself up for the next repetition, roll over and use your hands and elbows to help you back up to the starting position.
- Repeat 6 times.

REGULAR PUSH-UP (CHEST, SHOULDERS, AND ARMS)

- This move offers the most resistance and should be attempted after you've mastered the knee push-up or have progressed your wall push-up to fairly close to the ground.

- Begin in a high plank position with your entire body parallel to the floor. Place your palms firmly on the ground, directly under your shoulders. Your arms should be straight. Ground your toes into the floor to stabilize your body. Tighten your abs and flatten your back so your entire body is neutral and straight.
- Begin to lower your body toward the floor. This is the eccentric part of the move. Keep your back flat and let your chest graze the floor. Don't let your hips dip or stick out at any point during the move; your body should remain in a straight line from head to toe.
- Lower the knees to the ground and then return to the starting position however you like. This is 1 repetition.
- Repeat for 6 repetitions.

To increase resistance: Perform this move wearing a weight vest, or even with a small child seated on your back.

Back

GYM EQUIVALENTS: LAT PULLDOWN CABLE OR MACHINE, ASSISTED PULL-UP MACHINE, SEATED ROW, BENT-OVER ROW

Inverted Row

- Wrap a resistance band or heavy strap evenly around a very sturdy pole, tree, or banister. Grip the ends of the band/strap in each hand, elbows bent, and fists held in toward your low rib cage.
- Tighten your core and eccentrically lower your chest away from the support by slowly straightening your arms to the count of 10. Use the band to help you, and keep your body as stiff as possible.
- Once your arms are straight, that is 1 repetition. Repeat 6 times.

To increase resistance: Increase the angle of your body to the floor (the more parallel your body becomes to the floor, the greater the resistance) and use less resistance on the bands.

Resistance Band Row

- Sit on the floor or exercise mat with your legs outstretched in front of you. Loop the middle of a resistance band around the bottoms of your feet. Grip each handle with your hands. If you can't sit on the ground with your legs outstretched, place a folded towel or blanket under your hips. This provides the height to maintain a neutral low back. As an alternative, you can perform this move seated in a chair and the band around a sturdy pole or bannister.
- Begin to hinge forward at the waist and hold the handles with your elbows bent and against your low ribs.
- Then as you sit up straight, pull the handles back until they are next to your side and your elbows are behind you. Squeeze your shoulder blades together and keep your chest up.
- Eccentrically and slowly straighten your arms to the count of 10.
- Repeat 6 times.
- To increase resistance: Use both hands to pull the handles back, and then hold both handles in one hand for the eccentric portion of the movement. You can also add another band, decrease the length of the band between your hands, or use a band that offers greater tension.

Resistance Band Lat Pull-Down

- Secure a resistance band around the middle of a sturdy support point, such as a bannister. This point needs to be above the level of your head during the movement.
- Grip a handle with each hand and kneel down on the floor or exercise mat, 3 to 4 feet from the support structure. This move can also be done seated. Keep your back straight, head straight, shoulders down, and arms pointed toward the support structure with your palms facing forward.
- Pull the handles down and out to the sides until your hands are even with your chin. Eccentrically and slowly return to the starting position.

- Repeat 6 times.
- To increase resistance: Use both hands to pull the bands down, and then hold both ends of the band in one hand for the eccentric portion of the movement. You can also add another band, decrease the length of the band between your hands, or use a band that offers greater tension.

Negative Pull-Ups (Back)

- Find something sturdy to hang from. It should be no lower than your chin if you are standing on the ground and no higher than your chin if you are standing on a chair. Common options include jungle gyms/swing sets, tree branches, or an inexpensive pull-up bar you've installed in your home.
- Stand on the ground or on a chair so that your chin is slightly above the apparatus you are going to hang from.
- With your arms slightly wider than shoulder-width apart, put your hands on top of the apparatus. Grip it as tightly as you can. Stick your chest out and squeeze your shoulder blades together.
- Using a firm grip, start to bend your legs so that you begin to hang with bent elbows from the apparatus. The more you bend your legs, the more challenging it will be to hang on.
- While you are hanging on, your back and arms will get tired, and you will slowly lower down until your arms are fully extended. If your arms fully extend in less than 10 seconds, you are using your legs too little. If your arms fully extend in more than 10 seconds, you are using your legs too much. While your arms are extending and you are lowering down, keep your shoulders back, keep your chest out, look up, and keep your arms as even with your torso as possible—that is, do not let your arms creep out in front of you.
- After your arms have fully extended, simply stand up to get your chin back above the bar.
- Repeat 6 more times without resting.

- To increase resistance: Use your legs less and less by bending your knees more. To add even more resistance, add weight to your hips by looping a chain around your hips or hanging weights from a weight belt.

Shoulders/Arms
GYM EQUIVALENTS: SHOULDER-PRESS MACHINE, DUMBBELL SHOULDER PRESS

<u>Banded Shoulder Press</u>

- Stand with a staggered stance, one foot forward. Place the middle of an exercise band under the arch of your front foot. This can also be done seated on a chair.
- Hold both ends of the band in each hand with your thumbs near your armpits. Make a fist and keep your wrists from bending or flopping. Push straight up until your elbows are straight.
- Transfer both ends of the band to one hand and slowly, to the count of 10, bend the elbow until your fist is back to the starting position.
- Repeat 6 times per arm.
- To increase resistance: Double up on bands or choose a band that offers greater tension.

<u>Inverted Push-Up</u>

- Set up in a high plank position on the floor or exercise mat. Your arms should be straight and your hands should be shoulder-width apart.
- Lift up your hips so that your body forms an upside down V, and come up on your toes. Bend your elbows slowly, to the count of 10, and lower your upper body until the top of your head nearly touches the floor. That is 1 repetition.
- Lower your knees to the floor or walk your feet toward your hands to exit the position. Set yourself back up in the inverted position and repeat 6 times.

- To increase resistance: Raise the height of your hips by either
  walking your feet in more toward your hands or placing your
  feet on something higher.

Caution: This movement should not be performed without approval from
your doctor if you have high blood pressure or glaucoma.

SANE INTERVALS

Most people know how to pedal an upright stationary bike, so getting started with
SANE interval training has a smaller learning curve than eccentric exercise. You
will see a lot of benefits from doing this once a week, even before you are an eccentric exercise expert.

- Hop onto an upright stationary bike on which you can adjust
  resistance. (Do not use a recumbent bike—the type that looks
  like a recliner.)
- Warm up by pedaling at a moderate pace with moderate
  resistance—for about 3 minutes.
- Increase the bike's resistance so that you can pedal only by
  standing up on the pedals and pushing down on them as
  hard as you can. Apply plenty of resistance, but not so that you
  are twisting and contorting your body to move the pedals.
  On the other hand, without enough resistance, you will have
  trouble keeping your feet on the pedals, and you won't feel much
  effort at all.
- Pedal hard like that for 30 seconds—as if you're running from
  a tiger. If you can pedal for longer than 30 seconds, increase the
  resistance until you cannot.
- Rest for 2 minutes by decreasing the resistance and pedaling
  moderately.
- Repeat three more sets of 30 seconds' pedaling hard paired with
  2 minutes' active recovery.

Resistance is important here. You're not doing SANE interval training
if you get on an upright stationary bike and flail around uncontrollably for

30 seconds. Sounds silly, but that is exactly what will happen if you don't add enough resistance.

Moving your body very quickly will eventually lead to an injury. However, by adding resistance, you can move at a normal, controllable, and safe rate, while working as forcefully as you possibly can. SANE interval training is not about moving faster. It's about moving more resistance.

When working out on a stationary bicycle, proper form is important. Adjust the seat height correctly. If your seat is too low or too high, your legs won't pedal efficiently, and you could place undue stress on your knee or hip joint. Find the correct seat height by placing one of the pedals in the fully lowered position. Sit on the bike and extend your leg to the pedal, making sure there's a slight bend in your knee. If not, readjust the seat accordingly.

Sit up straight, too. Keep your shoulder blades squeezed down and back and bring your belly button back toward your spine. Grip the bike handlebars lightly.

Keep in mind that you don't have to use an upright stationary bike, but you do need to use a low-impact machine such as an elliptical trainer that will provide enough resistance to exhaust yourself in 30 seconds without having to move quickly. This means you cannot do SANE intervals safely on a treadmill, because there is no way to add resistance without increasing speed or risk.

As with the eccentric exercises, there is a learning curve to SANE interval training. Start off with less resistance, focus on proper form, and concentrate on using your legs. Then work up from there. When you do that, you'll experience "jelly legs" and an empowering heart-pounding feeling. Both are signs that you're working out smartly and SANEly.

WHEN TO START SANE ACTIVITY: THE PRACTICE PRINCIPLE

Moving your muscles in an eccentric fashion is probably brand-new to you. There is a learning curve and a need for practice time prior to you jumping in. If your goal was to run a marathon, you likely wouldn't attempt to run 26 miles on day one. The same applies here. When you perform new exercises, or challenge your body in a new way, your body responds by increasing its ability to cope with the new load. This is called *neuromuscular adaptation*. You can improve your body's physiological response to SANE activity through practice. So I want you to practice eccentric moves before you even begin doing the SANE eccentrics for 10 minutes a week. Here's how:

- Get a feel for the resistance of a move, particularly when using resistance bands or your own body weight (as in push-ups), especially if you have never done resistance training or eccentric training in the past.
- Practice both the lifting (concentric) and lowering (eccentric) phases of the movements. Avoid any jerking, twisting, or quick moves.
- Follow the simple rule of lowering the resistance at a rate twice as long as it took to raise it.
- Don't add heavy resistance to your eccentric workouts the first 2 weeks of the 21-Day Plan; just practice the motions.
- During the last week of the 21-Day Plan, start the eccentric workout with enough resistance. Because you're used to the movements, you can push hard.
- Write down how you feel after training eccentrically. (See the section below on keeping an exercise journal.)

YOUR WEEKLY SANE WORKOUT

Here is a look at your week (begin in week 3 of the 21-Day Plan), and you're going to love it. You're investing only 20 minutes a week in your body's development—which ensures you are "exercising to live" instead of "living to exercise." Call me crazy, but I don't think most people want to be remembered for their abs, but instead for their contributions to their family, friends, and the world. How you eat and how you move should serve you, not the other way around. Here's how you'll do that:

Day 1: 10 minutes of SANE eccentric training
Day 2: Relax and recover
Day 3: Relax and recover
Day 4: 10 minutes of SANE interval training
Day 5: Relax and recover

Day 6: Relax and recover

Day 7: Relax and recover

Think of your SANE workout as the most efficient way to empower and energize your new lifestyle. Twenty minutes for a transformed 20 years (and more). Not a bad deal.

ONCE YOU MASTER AT-HOME ECCENTRICS, JOIN AN INEXPENSIVE GYM

At some point, you will get into such great shape that your body weight, resistance bands, or weight vests no longer provide enough resistance to work all your muscle fibers. So, if you want to improve your fitness, you'll need to exercise eccentrically on machines at a gym.

Keep in mind that the most basic and inexpensive gym will do the trick. You need only the four machines, namely a sled leg press, chest press machine, lat pulldown machine (or rowing machine), and a shoulder-press machine. At a gym, too, you also have a large selection of dumbbells, barbells, kettlebells, and other free weights.

However, protect yourself from the complexity that many gyms try to sell you. The more complex a gym tries to make exercise sound, the faster you should run in the other direction. Actual fitness experts know that 99 percent of the population can achieve all their goals using a leg-press type of movement, a pull-up or row movement, and chest- and shoulder-press movements. Unless you are an elite athlete, everything else is marketing. The person selling it to you will make it sound wondrous, but it is generally unnecessary for everyone except the salesperson.

Most gyms will give you a tour of the facilities and equipment before you join, so it's easy to determine whether it meets your needs. In lieu of joining a gym or health club, look into the YMCA or community centers—all of which are generally more cost-effective.

SANE ACTIVITY TIPS

You are going to get phenomenal results by working out SANEly—activating more muscle fibers through brief, infrequent workouts that exercise your muscles slowly and eccentrically. Here are the top four tips our most successful members use to supercharge the setpoint-lowering effects of SANE activity:

1. Before You Begin: Prepare your body to work out. Always warm up first to prevent injury and to help you perform the movements more effectively. An ideal warm-up involves doing enough movement to elevate your body temperature—about 3 minutes of moderate pedaling on a stationary bike or a short, brisk walk. After you've got some blood flowing, it is fine to do some light muscle stretches, with no long holds and an emphasis on moving your joints through their full pain-free range of motion.

2. During Your Workout: Don't hold your breath during your eccentrics. Breathe freely and as much as you need to help you control the resistance. If your face gets all red and you are sweating profusely and huffing and puffing, that is something to be proud of, not embarrassed. All that effort means big results when it comes to permanently lowering your setpoint weight. If you need to take a break between repetitions or sets, note it in your exercise journal. Decreasing the amount of time needed to rest can also count toward measuring your forward progress.

3. After Your Workout: After a workout, your muscles require an immediate supply of amino acids to start the rebuilding process. This is an excellent time to consume a SANE smoothie made with clean whey protein. It is rich in leucine, which as you'll recall is essential for muscle development because it turns on the process of muscle protein synthesis (MPS) and supplies critical building blocks for muscle protein.

This also helps to soothe delayed-onset muscle soreness (DOMS). Eccentric exercise will make your muscles sore, and it typically begins to develop 12 to 24 hours after you've exercised. It's nothing to worry about, though. It's a sign you've deeply worked all your muscle fibers and is only a side effect of the muscle repair taking place. If DOMS bothers you, apply an ice pack to the tender areas. But one of the best ways to reduce its severity is to properly warm up prior to exercising. Then be patient. You will get less and less sore over time.

4. Between Workouts: Increase circulation and decrease stiffness by doing light activity such as stretching and gently moving your joints through their full range of motion. Use a foam roller, if you wish. Though not required, this is an exercise tool that helps alleviate any tension or tightness within muscles.

You can target your legs, hips, upper back, and other parts of the body for a great self-massage between workouts. A foam roller works by breaking up soft tissue tightness and increasing circulation to help with movement throughout the body. It can also be used to increase circulation and release tension before workouts or after your workout as a part of a cooldown.

Will SANE Workouts Make Me Hungry?

No. Short, intense exercises like those in the SANE workout are unique because they suppress the hunger hormone ghrelin and lower cortisol.

In a study published in *Medicine & Science in Sports & Exercise*, people who did SANE-type interval training on a stationary bike ate the equivalent of 120 calories less during their postworkout meals than those who pedaled continuously at a moderate pace (Sim et al. 2015). Exercising did not increase appetite in the interval trainers!

Where traditional exercise drives you to eat inSANE foods, your body reacts to SANE workouts by curbing your hunger. It just keeps getting better and better!

KEEP A SANE EXERCISE JOURNAL

An exercise journal or log is a helpful tool to help you reach your goals as quickly and efficiently as possible. With a journal, you can track your progress and have a written record of how your body is changing for the better. Some suggestions:

- Use something convenient and portable—something that is easy to carry around and keep in your pocket while you're working out. This could be a small notebook or even the notes function on your smartphone.
- Write down the exercises you did, the repetitions, and the resistance you used. Also, describe your mood and energy levels on any given workout day.

- Every so often, look at your previous entries to psych yourself up, because you're getting stronger, using more resistance, and performing better week by week.
- After just a few weeks of exercising, ask yourself how you feel compared to how you felt before you started to exercise. Are some exercises easier to do now? Are you feeling more energy throughout the day? Are you sleeping better? Record your answers.

When you can see and feel improvements in your weight and health, it can be a great motivator to keep improving and getting stronger.

SANE activity is a wonderful and required complement to a SANE lifestyle, but, much in the way exercise cannot undo the damage done to our respiratory system by smoking, the same is true for the damage done to our metabolic system by inSANE foods. By focusing primarily on eating more but smarter, and secondarily on exercising less but smarter, you can simplify your life, while enjoying long-term results you never thought possible.

SANE Points

- Perform a routine of four eccentric resistance exercises for 10 minutes on one day and SANE interval training for 10 minutes on another day. Allow enough time for rest and recovery, and always warm up prior to exercising.
- Focus on making some improvement, no matter how small, each time you do a SANE workout.
- Enjoy a SANE smoothie with clean whey protein after your workouts in order to support muscle repair and development.
- SANEly manage muscle soreness or tightness with adequate rest and the use of a foam roller.
- Avoid overexercising; it leads to potential health problems and cravings for inSANE foods.
- Add restorative activities into your exercise program in order to manage stress and clear stress hormones.
- Track your progress with an exercise journal, and congratulate yourself on your amazing accomplishments.

PART 5

SANE MIND-SET

CHAPTER 13

Love Yourself Slim

Change is hard. You probably know you need to make changes in your life, but you may feel stuck. The secret to getting unstuck and feeling back in control of your health is to discover methods that make lasting change instantaneous. Of course, you won't lose all the pounds in an instant (that's not how your biology works), but in an instant your perception can change, immediately ending this *struggle* and making an almost unimaginably bright future infinitely more achievable (that *is* how SANE psychology works).

It might be hard to wrap your ahead around this concept now, but by the time you finish this and the next chapter, you'll have a whole new mind-set that will make achieving your new body so much easier. For example, think about a woman who smoked most of her life and is addicted to nicotine, the third most addictive substance in the world, and finds out she's pregnant. She stops smoking instantly. How is instantly changing behavior linked to a chemical addiction possible?

Once you get that moment of clarity—boom—you "get it"; there is no going back. Please believe it can happen for you. No matter how much you have struggled in the past, when you give yourself permission to take on a SANE mind-set, you will experience these types of breakthrough moments. Your perception of food, fitness, your body, and even your "self" will transform, and you will achieve your long-term weight and health goals without worry or struggle.

So why hasn't this happened to you yet? Until now, you haven't been given the right tools. You see, it's not just about "what to eat" or "how to exercise." If you have ever struggled with sticking to a plan consistently over the long run, breaking old habits, dealing with cravings and emotional eating, engaging in self-sabotaging behaviors, or simply staying motivated, then you are missing the key tool our most successful members call "the SANE mind-set."

Trying to change how you eat, exercise, and live without a SANE mind-set is like getting on the freeway and attempting to change lanes without a steering wheel. You may get lucky and get where you want to go sometimes, but most likely you will veer off course and get into a wreck. It doesn't matter if you have a stack of maps, or the best GPS system in the world, or even a professional driving instructor sitting next to you, if you do not have the tools needed to put all that *information* into *action*, you will not consistently get where you want to go. The instant you give yourself permission to adopt the SANE mind-set, you will be able to put all the *information* you are learning into *action* effortlessly.

If you have ever felt like you "know what to do" but struggle with "doing what you know" in today's insane world, then what you are about to learn will have a dramatic impact on your life, your setpoint weight, your health, and your overall happiness. Why? Because practically every "weight-loss" program on the planet is missing the vital ingredients for success that you are learning here. You can't *will* your speeding mind to change course any more than you can *will* your racing car to change course.

There is an alternative path with amazing psychological tools that work *with* your brain rather than against it—tools proven by modern psychology you won't find in any weight-loss program, anywhere. You have learned how to work *with* your biology with a completely different model for eating and caring for your body; now you're going to learn how to *work* with your psychology. Much like you can instantly and permanently change the direction of even a massive truck once you put your hands on the wheel, you will be able to instantly change the direction of massive health challenges once we put your hands on your wheel with the SANE mind-set.

It begins with the story you tell yourself about your life and the words you use to talk to yourself. As you read these chapters, keep this question in mind: What story am I telling myself about my weight and my body? Is it true? Really, is it true? And then actually write out an answer to that question. Honestly. Listen to what you are saying to yourself, ask "Is that true?" and start writing.

Start considering the possibility that you can rewrite your story and rewire the way you talk to yourself. Instead of struggling with bad habits, you can easily replace them with positive, health-promoting habits that lower your set-point weight automatically. You never have to look at the scale again. Instead you are looking in the mirror into the confident eyes of a new slim, vibrant you, with more than enough energy to do all the things you've always wanted to do. You genuinely love yourself, and the years of shame and guilt are sinking into far-off memories. You never feel bad about the choices you make. You have control. Effortless control. Finally.

When you reshape the story that you tell yourself and change the conversation that's going on in your head, you will experience positive results that no food list could ever match. The *only* path to permanent weight loss requires that you believe in yourself and that you love yourself, so on these pages, I want to give you the clinically proven tools to do just that. It's time to create a new empowering story, and that is exactly what you and I will do.

No matter what the voice in your head is saying right now, or what your story is, you absolutely do deserve to look and feel your best. When the voice in your head is telling you the right story, filled with truth, appreciation, and confidence, you will find that consistently making SANE choices, and subsequently lowering your setpoint and then permanently losing weight, becomes almost effortless. If you are ready for that turning point in your life, the one that leads to permanent and lasting weight loss, then let's get started.

PROGRESS VERSUS PERFECTION

The number-one psychological secret to lowering your setpoint weight is letting go of the pressure to be perfect. In fact, the surest way to struggle is to seek perfection. It is essential that you shift your focus to "make progress" and let go of "be perfect."

The idea of "I need to be perfect" makes change impossible because it robs you of the belief that you can change. Deep down, you know that "perfect," especially when it comes to how you eat or how you look, is literally impossible.

What does "perfect" even mean? And have you ever met a perfect person? I wrote the book on SANE, and I am not perfectly SANE every second of the day. I don't expect you to be perfect. I don't want you to be perfect! And I need you to not expect nor want YOU to be perfect. It's not a realistic or helpful expectation.

Consider a different mind-set. Imagine if you believed the following: "What if each day I got 1 percent better? Then, in 100 days, I'd be 100 percent better." It's the simple math of sustainable change, and 100 days are the blink of an eye when you think of all the time you've spent struggling with your weight. The best part is that a 1 percent improvement is easy when you use SANE tools, while trying to be 100 percent better overnight is a recipe for disappointment. If that has ever happened to you, you are not the only one. You are not alone anymore, because together we are going to change that. Starting today, you are going to be courageously consistent at getting a little better each day. You are going to stack small, sustainable success on top of small, sustainable success and your setpoint will plummet.

For example, here's what a day could look like when you focus on progress, getting 1 percent better, and not perfection. You start your day by making a SANE green smoothie. Just this simple action shows you that you are worth loving and that you deserve to start your day with the most convenient and optimal source of nutrition imaginable. Besides the cascade of feel-good emotions after your SANE smoothie, you have already enjoyed 5 servings of non-starchy vegetables, along with 1 serving of nutrient-dense protein, so your body and mind feel satisfied and full of energy.

You then effortlessly make another small step by skipping your usual sugar-filled mocha latte supreme—not because you will yourself to but because you have so much natural energy from your SANE smoothie that you don't want it. In fact, thanks to all that extra energy, you decide to take a walk in the park for some restorative activity, while enjoying the sun and the nature around you. Inspired by your earlier successes, at dinner you swap out your usual soda for a refreshing glass of lemon water. That's a lot of progress in just one day!

The best part is these small changes have a compound effect, just like earning interest in your bank account. It's not the size of the change that matters; it's being able to stick with it, enjoyably and consistently. You are making small, meaningful changes toward your goals. Not only is this effective, but it also makes you feel great, which gives you the motivation to take the next small step, which then makes you feel even better—and wow, before you know it, you are somewhere you never thought possible. You have begun to rewrite the story of your life.

Write this down and post it everywhere you can (desk, car, fridge, etc.): "Nobody's perfect. I am making progress."

BREAK THE CYCLE OF SHAME

When you require "perfection" to feel successful, you will constantly feel ashamed. Shame is a powerful emotion. In fact, renowned psychiatrist, physician, and researcher Sir David R. Hawkins, MD, PhD, has found that shame is the most debilitating of all emotions. It literally weakens you more than any other emotion you could possibly feel.

This is because shame is the intensely painful feeling of being fundamentally flawed and therefore being unworthy of anything positive. It is the root cause of many struggles in your life, particularly with your weight, body image, and self-esteem. Even worse, feeling shame can cause you to feel ashamed about feeling shame. That leads to a vicious and setpoint-skyrocketing downward shame spiral. Until we break you free from this insane cycle of shame, no food or fitness plan will give you the experience of life that you are after.

What does the insane shame cycle look like in real life? Take a situation like a weekend binge on sweets. Shame says, "You are a bad person who never has self-control!" But the objective truth is actually a little different: "I ate a lot of cookies, which moves me further away from my goals." This may sound like a small distinction, but understanding the difference is essential. It is the difference between thinking you are a bad person and thinking that a specific *action* is bad.

When you feel ashamed about who you are as a person, how motivated do you feel to make SANEr choices and to take care of yourself with the love and respect you truly deserve? Compare that to knowing that you made an isolated mistake and will do better in the future. It's the difference between a slight bump in the road and the *end* of the road.

Shame is setpoint poison because it attacks the part of you that believes you can create lasting change. How can you ever make positive changes if you believe you are inherently bad, flawed, wrong? If "you" are the problem, then "you" have no hope of solving the problem. Ever hear the old saying "Wherever you go, there you are"?

The truth is: You are not the problem. The problem is always something external, a choice that was made or a habit that has become hard to overcome. To put it more simply: The problem is the problem!

This is especially true about food. In my own research and working with clients for more than 15 years, I have found that everything that encourages shame about food is guaranteed to make you fat, sick, and sad. And unfortunately, shame involving what people eat or do not eat is rampant and causes a condition I call FOF, or the Fear of Food. It's time to take back your power and toss shame in the trash along with the tools that cause it: your scale, food scales, calorie counters, and all that nonsense.

Shame and Moral Licensing

One of the ways shame-based labeling of foods and behaviors as "good" or "bad" causes you to sabotage your goals is called "moral licensing." This term describes a pattern where even "good" behavior has setpoint-elevating results. For example, have you ever said to yourself, "I had a bunch of great workouts this week, so I'm going to splurge on pizza and desserts this weekend"? In other words, rewarding yourself for something "good" with inSANE foods that elevate your setpoint.

Now that you know food is more than just calories, you can see just how counterproductive this is. "Rewarding" yourself for exercising by eating a cupcake is like "rewarding" yourself for exercising by smoking a pack of cigarettes. Exercising off calories doesn't "cancel out" the setpoint-elevating damage of the cupcake any more than exercising off calories cancels out the cancer-causing damage of smoking. The end result is that shame-based moral licensing—that is, doing "bad" to reward "good"—at best leads you to take one step forward, and two steps back.

The "What the Hell" Effect

Unfortunately, the setpoint-elevating impact of shame gets even worse because it triggers what scientists call the "what-the-hell effect," the cycle of indulgence, regret, and greater indulgence.

For example: "Well, that doughnut I ate for breakfast messed up my 'points' for the day, so might as well make this a 'bad' day and eat pizza for lunch and ice cream for dinner." Then tomorrow rolls around and the internal dialog happens: "Since yesterday was so 'bad,' what the hell, might as well forget the whole week." And a "bad" meal becomes a "bad" day becomes a "bad" week becomes a "bad" month becomes a "bad" year becomes a "bad" decade becomes diabesity and an elevated setpoint!

So how do you prevent this vicious cycle? The most important move you can make is to recognize when you start moralizing eating or anything related to your weight or health. What do you think about who you are as a person when you eat SANEly? Do you immediately think of ways to "reward" yourself for being so "good"? What do you think about who you are as a person when you eat inSANEly? Do you immediately become self-critical and beat yourself up for being "bad"?

The antidote to this insanity is to shift into a mind-set of self-compassion instead. Self-compassion is treating yourself with the same kindness and care that you would extend to someone that you love. In a multipart study published in the *Journal of Social and Clinical Psychology*, Duke University researchers instructed a group of body-conscious women to eat a Dunkin' Donuts doughnut (Adams and Leary 2007). After eating the doughnut, half of the women were given a message of self-compassion and self-forgiveness, encouraging them to not be harsh on themselves for indulging. The other group of women did not receive this message and were left to their own self-critical thinking.

In the next part of the study, the women were then served bowls filled with candy, including Reese's and Skittles, and were invited to eat as little or as much of the candy as they wanted to. The women who were given the self-compassion, self-forgiveness message ate less than half as much candy as the women who didn't get that message. That's the huge difference self-compassion and self-forgiveness can cause. They help shut off the stream of shame and guilt and prevent "what the hell" type thinking to lead to inSANE choices and downward spirals.

Think of a time in your life when you felt the "what-the-hell" effect. What was going on in your brain then? Were you being self-critical? What was the little story you told yourself? Building awareness is the first step to making a change in this vicious cycle. Beating yourself up for having these thoughts won't change anything. Instead, recognize when these thoughts are present and start to develop an awareness of what triggers them. When they happen, take three minutes to write them down and then ask yourself: "What would I say to a friend who experienced the same setback?"

Keep in mind, too, that your "setback" is not the end of the world. Setbacks are normal and expected parts of life that everyone will encounter. They don't define you as a person, nor do they mean you're a failure. Focus on self-compassion—responding to yourself with kindness, both through words and actions, whenever possible.

Another part of being self-compassionate is to take the shame, judgment, and fear out of food and fitness. To lower your setpoint as effectively as possible, instead of putting "good" and "bad" labels on every food or action, focus on what you can learn from what happened. If you eat a doughnut, ask yourself what led up to your decision and how you could make a SANEr choice the next time you are in that situation. This is the "progress vs. perfection" mind-set in action. It helps you avoid "bad" causing "bad" (what-the-hell effect) and "good" causing "bad" (moral licensing).

The Solution to Shame Cycling

You are a miracle. Seriously. I am a science guy and can tell you that there is no scientific explanation for how you came to be. You are rarer than the rarest diamond. That's not "woo woo." That is a mathematical fact. And it's essential you *know* that you are a miracle, because to break free from shame, you must be able to recognize that shame is a lie. Nothing you do—especially nothing about how you look, eat, or exercise—can strip you of your worth. I need you to really get that. You have tremendous worth no matter what you do or how you look.

Therefore, if your mind starts to send you shame signals, you must recognize that those are lies. Think about it like this: When you look at an optical illusion, your brain tells you something you know isn't true. Shame is an "emotional illusion." Once you can see that, you escape from the setpoint-elevating effects of shame in an instant.

The first step to this freedom from shame is understanding the three characteristics of shame: personal, pervasive, and permanent—or the three poison Ps. In other words, shame is personal because it is about you, the *person*. It's *pervasive* because it affects all areas of your life. Finally, because it's about who you are, it is *permanent*. For example, say Jane eats a piece of birthday cake at her son's birthday party. If she feels shame, it's because she thinks something like this: "I (personal) always (permanent) mess everything up (pervasive)." Compare that to this reaction, which would not have triggered shame: "That party was awkward (not personal, not pervasive). I will not stand right next to the cake next year (not permanent)."

Can Jane accurately conclude that she always messes up everything because she ate a piece of cake? She ate a piece of cake. That's it. If you have made choices in the past that did not move you closer toward your goals, here's what that means:

"You have made choices in the past that did not move you closer toward your goals." Period. It doesn't take away from your worth. It doesn't tell you anything about every area of your life. It can't tell you anything about your future.

To start replacing shame with self-compassion, try this: On a sheet of paper or in a journal, list three areas or situations in which you felt shame. These can be about what you ate or how much you ate. It may be about how you feel about your body. It may even be about how you think others see you. As always, there are no right or wrong answers. Just go with the first three things that come to mind.

Now pick one of those three. Choose one that holds the most emotion for you. Write down what shame said about you in that situation or is even saying right now. Identify the personal, persuasive, and permanent aspects of what shame is saying. Can you see how those are lies? Directly challenge each of the three poison Ps with "Is that true? Really, is it objectively true?" Or if you are really struggling with shame, you may find it more helpful to imagine someone you love feeling the way you feel now. How would you respond to the lies shame is telling about *them*? Write it down. The key is to catch shame harassing you and lying to you, and defending yourself because you know you deserve better because you know you are a miracle.

Leave Behind "Scale Shame"

Do you have a scale in your home? Do you use it regularly? Every time you step on the scale, consider your motivation. What is the point of weighing yourself? What does your weight tell you about what's happening to your setpoint? Nothing. The number on the scale shows you the effect of gravity on your body, and that's all, and that's not helpful for lowering your setpoint. So what is the real reason you are stepping on that scale? If the number was 5 pounds more than it was yesterday, how would you feel? Do you hear shame's voice start chattering away? This just makes you feel stuck, overwhelmed, inadequate, and judged, inside and out.

Basing your value and worth on that number you see on the scale is a recipe for feelings of shame, guilt, and judgment. Please give yourself permission to break free from this insanity. Weighing yourself tells you *nothing* about what's happening with your setpoint and is therefore useless for long-term weight loss. In fact, it's counterproductive because the scale encourages you to starve yourself, which increases your setpoint. Continually weighing yourself doesn't work. If it did, it would have worked already.

What I suggest is that at the very least you hide your scale so you won't be tempted to use it. What I'd prefer is that you have a "set myself free from shame" ceremony where you destroy or dispose of your scale (and ideally video record it or take a picture so you remember and can share them with me[11]). Getting rid of your scale is a concrete and memorable way to prove to yourself that you are giving up shame and self-sabotage and embracing self-care and love. It proves that you are done with focusing on theoretical future fantasies that feel impossible, and instead you are focused on the realistic simple steps you can take today to progress toward your long-term goals.

THE SANE WAY TO SET AND ACHIEVE GOALS

All the diets you have tried in the past didn't effectively lower your setpoint. This is because they focused you on *negative* goals (do *not* eat too much fat, do *not* eat too many calories, do *not* eat too many points, do *not* eat after 6:00 p.m.) instead of *positive* goals (eat more non-starchy vegetables, eat more nutrient-dense protein, eat more whole-food fats). At best, negative goals make success harder; at worst they make it impossible. Here's why: When you tell your brain "don't do something," your brain responds by hyperfocusing on that thing. What else is it supposed to do? If your ancestors were out hunting and told themselves, "Don't get eaten by a tiger," what is the only thing their brain can do to help them? Put tigers at the top of their mind!

You can see this in your own life anytime you've felt nervous and found that

---

[11] Please email your scale liberation videos and pictures to Service@SANESolution.com and we'll send you back a neat surprise!

the more you tell yourself "Don't be nervous," the more nervous you became! The more your brain hears "Don't be nervous," the more it hyperfocuses on things that could make you nervous. Ironically, the harder you try *not* to do something the more likely it becomes.

The same thing happens with food. Have you ever tried not to think about a certain food? What immediately happens? You think more and more about that food. In other words, when you tell yourself, "Don't think about X" or "Avoid X," it's like your brain hires a private investigator to be constantly looking for X everywhere. Want to make it as hard as possible to avoid sugar? Tell yourself, "No sugar." What is your brain going to help you see everywhere and think about all the time? Sugar.

To get your goals working for you—rather than against you—make sure they focus you on *pursuing the positive* rather than *attacking the negative*. This approach empowers your brain to keep what you want at the top of your mind, and you effortlessly find opportunities to lower your setpoint everywhere. Instead of experiencing life as an exhausting slog through a minefield of things to avoid, you experience life as a treasure hunt with setpoint-lowering delights wherever you look. For instance, you go to a party and don't even see the inSANE foods because your brain automatically focuses on the sliced veggies, meat, and, look, there's even some shrimp!

This approach is awesome because it works *with* your brain—rather than against it—and thus makes reaching your goals much easier. In this SANE approach to goal-setting, you are going to be adding positive strategies rather than depriving yourself. By setting goals that *pursue the positive* rather than *attacking the negative*, you will get better results *and* have a more enjoyable time getting there!

Bite-Sized Success

Have you ever come up with a big goal, and after only a few days, you felt overwhelmed and possibly paralyzed, thinking to yourself, "How in the heck am I going to get from here all the way to there?"

As much as self-help gurus tell us to create massive goals and then plaster them all over a vision board, new research from Harvard, Northwestern, and the University of Pennsylvania show why this doesn't work. While massive far-off future goals sound sexy and wonderful, the approach isn't supported by science. If you have ever set a massive goal and didn't reach it, you didn't fail. That approach failed you!

In fact, modern science shows that most often these far-off future goals *decrease* your chances of success. I know this sounds crazy after all the "goals gone wild" messages you've heard, but think about it: How has that advice worked out for you so far? Are far-off future goals fun to set, then overwhelming within a week? They're almost like mental junk food—enjoyable in the moment, but because they have no substance, they leave you feeling worse after you come down from the initial high.

Results Goals versus Process Goals

If you tell yourself you are going to lose 100 pounds, that is a specific type of goal called a "results goal." The problem with results goals is that they focus on things you may not be able to control, and they take place in the future. A SANEr approach is to set process goals that deal with things you can control right now—for example, drinking a SANE smoothie with breakfast.

While small process goals you can achieve today may not seem sexy on the surface, I promise that achieving them consistently is the key to everything you want in life. The only thing you can control is your actions. So why focus on anything other than taking *positive* actions to lower your setpoint now? Look at it this way: If you achieve small process goals consistently—for example, eating one more serving of green veggies today than you did yesterday—you can't *help* but eventually get where you want to go.

Continuous progress today adds up to massive transformation over time—for two big reasons. First, you are hardwired to be a goal-completing biological machine. Even if they are small, checking things off your to-do list feels great. When you complete small daily process goals, you set yourself up to easily complete the next goal in front of you because you have positive thoughts and emotions driving you forward.

If you focus only on your future final goal weight, you never get to feel the excitement and joy of those small everyday wins. In fact, you'll experience the exact opposite. You'll only feel the anxiety and stress of "failing" at that "perfect" future goal repeatedly. You wake up and think, "Am I at my 'perfect' weight? No. Failure. How about now? No. Failure. Now?" You get the point.

Second, this SANEr approach simplifies any process into bite-sized pieces that are fun to complete. You only need to focus on the next bite-sized task, which is clear, tiny, and easy, and that's motivating. For example, let's suppose you decide to run a marathon. If you have never run a mile before, and you try to compete in a marathon on day one, that will not go well. Instead, if running a marathon was your goal, you would start small by first buying a pair of running shoes. The next day you'd walk around the block. The next day, you would do that twice. The next day, you would pick up the pace. And on and on. Checking a lot of things off your list and having fun doing it. By taking small steps consistently, eventually you develop the positive momentum to enter the race.

What you did was take a big results goal and then you broke it down into the smallest pieces possible that are under your control—that is, process goals. Since you are reading this book to learn how to lower your setpoint, let's take an example results goal of effortlessly weighing 160 pounds. This is a results goal that you can kind of control,[12] and you can break it down into small steps you can control completely. You are literally shaping your future with present action. Here are some sample steps to do this in your own life:

Write down that positive results goal of effortlessly weighing 160 pounds (or whatever a healthy goal weight is for your height). Like we talked about, always make sure when writing a goal that you pursue the positive. Effortlessly weighing 160 pounds is positive; it states what you want. Losing 30 pounds is negative; it states what you don't want.

Next, break that goal down into two categories of process goals: Action Steps and Consistency Steps. Action Steps are one-time actions while Consistency Steps are actions that get repeated with regularity—goals that you will want to do consistently over time.

Examples of Action Steps are:

Find a gym close to my home or buy a good blender so I can make SANE smoothies.

Spend a half hour clearing my kitchen of all inSANE food. (These are things you generally need to do only once.)

---

[12] You can't completely control your weight. For example, your height has a major impact on your weight and you have zero control over that.

Examples of Consistency Steps are:

> Go to the gym every Monday and Thursday.
> Blend a SANE smoothie with breakfast daily.
> Eat at least 2 servings of non-starchy vegetables with each meal.

Again, frame up your Action and Consistency Steps positively—around what you will do, not negatively around what you won't do or avoid.

See the difference and how it makes things so much easier to take on one step at a time?

I'll show you how to do this in more detail in your 21-Day Plan, but if you want a preview, you can get started by sitting down and thinking of as many little process goals—Action Steps and Consistency Steps—that you can take that will lead you to your main results goal. Then choose one small Action Step and Consistency Step you can do today to increase your self-esteem and easily check off the list and start the ball rolling.

Also, another goal-setting and motivating action you can do to move your health in a positive direction is to track your Action and Consistency Steps in a journal. Every morning, write the small actions you want to take for the day and cross them off with joy as you complete them.

At the risk of repeating myself, make sure that your goals *pursue the positive*. If you write down a goal to "drink one less soda a day," that is a process goal, yes, but it is still negative. A more effective approach is to say: Drink one more SANE smoothie a day. That way, you have set a process goal in which you pursue the positive.

THE SECRET SAUCE TO A LOWER SETPOINT: IMPLEMENTATION INTENTIONS

A little known but very powerful psychological "secret" to make your Action and Consistency Steps stick is a technique called *implementation intentions*. You already know how to take a results goal and break it down into process goals that include both Action Steps and Consistency Steps. Implementation intentions specify:

- The behavior you intend to take.
- The situation where/when you will take that behavior.
- The ways you will overcome obstacles to that behavior.

In other words, implementation intentions specify the what, when, and where—and are written in an if/when/then format. *If/when situation X happens, then I will do behavior Y to reach positive process goal Z.* Implementation intentions are extremely powerful. They have been proven in hundreds of studies to significantly increase the likelihood of achieving your goals.

Psychologists from the University of Manchester in Great Britain undertook a study to test whether implementation intentions could help with weight loss (Armitage et al. 2017). There were 216 people in the study. All were following healthier eating plans but only some of them used implementation intentions.

The participants instructed to use implementation intentions were given a worksheet where the left-hand side of the page contained common situations in which people feel tempted to eat, and on the right-hand side was a list of possible solutions. The participants were asked to select a situation on the left-hand side that applied to them personally and draw a line linking it to a solution on the right-hand side to form an implementation intention. An example in the study was: *If I am tempted to eat when I feel uncomfortable, then I will do something else instead of eating when I need to relax or deal with tension.*

After 6 months, the researchers followed up with everyone. Amazingly, the individuals who set implementation intentions lost nearly twice as much weight as the controls!

An earlier study, published in *Health Psychology* in 2007, produced similarly encouraging findings (Luszczynska et al. 2007). University of Sussex researchers in Great Britain enrolled 55 overweight or obese women in a program designed to evaluate the effectiveness of implementation intentions. The women were assigned to either an implementation intention group or a control group. Over the course of 2 months, the women who wrote implementation intentions lost twice as much weight as the control group. The researchers noted: "Among obese or overweight women participating in a commercial weight-loss program, those who learn to form implementation intentions can achieve greater weight reduction."

These studies suggest that you can nearly double the effectiveness of your process goals by creating and using implementation intentions. Really think about that for a moment. What else do you know of that costs nothing, has no negative side effects, can be done anywhere by anyone, and has been shown in studies to nearly double weight loss? I can't think of anything else either, and that's why I hope you will give yourself the gift of implementation intentions.

Getting Started with Implementation Intentions

Implementation intentions define when, where, and how you want to act on your goal. There are two different aspects you need to consider when you set them:

1. Identify the action that you're going to take to accomplish a certain goal, and when to take it.
2. Identify possible obstacles to goal-achievement, and how you'll manage them.

For example:

When I get up in the morning, I will immediately put on my sneakers and jacket and go for a 30-minute walk to increase my restorative activity during the week.

If it is raining on my walking days, I will put on a poncho before I go outside.

When I get home from work, I will immediately reheat and eat one of my batch-prepared SANE meals (even if I don't feel like it).

Before I leave for work, I will look to see if I have enough SANE groceries to cook. If I do not, then I will stop at the grocery store on my way home and pick up a rotisserie chicken and a pack of frozen veggies.

If I am hungry between meals, then I will get a SANE smoothie out of a container on the second shelf of the refrigerator and drink it.

Let's look at how to create your own implementation intentions. Remember the sequence: *If situation X happens, then I will do behavior Y to reach positive process goal Z.*

All you need to do is fill in these blanks here:

If/when _____ (situation X happens), then I will _____ (do behavior Y) to achieve _____ (positive process goal Z).

When you create implementation intentions, you plan the specific action that you are going to take to reach your process goals, and when and where you are going to carry out that action. You're also creating a plan on how you will move forward even when an obstacle might get in your way. Give this one a try: "When I finish reading this chapter, I will write down three implementation intentions to help me eat more non-starchy vegetables tomorrow." (See what I did there?)

Making progress without seeking perfection, breaking the shame cycle, setting positive process goals, and taking Action Steps and Consistency Steps framed up with implementation intentions will transform your life. Combine this proven psychological science of behavior change with the metabolic science you now know about eating and exercise, and you *will* get to where you want to go. You will lower your setpoint while upgrading the story you tell yourself about food and your body. You will begin to love yourself and gently make lasting changes that lead to permanent weight loss. You will leave behind the frustration of quick fixes, shame, guilt, and blame and the embarrassment and broken promises of all the diets that have failed you in the past. You will genuinely love yourself again, care for yourself again, and finally see the change you deserve in your life...for the rest of your life. You will be sane and SANE.

SANE Points

- Strive for progress, not perfection. This guarantees success.
- Break the cycle of shame, moral licensing, and the "what the hell" effect, by not putting "good" and "bad" labels on food or actions. Start focusing on whether your actions will get you closer to your goals, and genuinely forgive yourself. You are not the problem (the problem is the problem).
- When you focus on negative goals (what *not* to do), you are telling your brain to focus on the things you are trying to avoid. This is counterproductive. Pursue the positive rather than attacking the negative. With this simple mental switch, your brain works for you, instead of against you, and lasting change and success become almost effortless.
- Frame your goal-setting with positive process goals, broken down into Action Steps and Consistency Steps, and mentally rehearse them with implementation intentions—and you will succeed, perhaps even doubling your results.

CHAPTER 14

Simple Setpoint-Lowering Habits

Much of the success story you rewrite for yourself will come directly from your daily habits. In fact, habits control more than 90 percent of what you do every day, automatically. This means that when you create positive habits, you create positive change, automatically.

Let's look at a real-life example of how habit change slims your waistline while expanding your wallet. Consider the habit of drinking a glass or two of fruit juice every day. This doesn't seem like much, but if you cut out this habit, what would happen? First, you would instantly consume about 50 fewer grams of sugar each day. With this tiny change, you will almost effortlessly eat 40 fewer pounds of sugar each year. To put that in perspective, the average 4-year-old weighs 40 pounds. That's a lot less hormonally damaging sugar with very little effort.

Second, you will save money. Let's say each glass of juice costs $.40. That's $.80 a day, or a total of $292 a year. Over a decade, that adds up to $2,920. I don't know about you, but an extra $2,920 in my pocket while watching belly fat disappear sounds pretty good to me.

Finally, and this is where the real power of creating new habits and positive behaviors shows up: Imagine if instead of two glasses of sugar-heavy fruit juice, you made a SANE smoothie. You basically substituted a setpoint-elevating habit for a setpoint-lowering habit. Now you are enjoying healing and slimming fiber, vitamins, and minerals; saving money; and effortlessly eating 40 fewer pounds of sugar each year without any deprivation or willpower.

Do you see how one small change in daily habits can have a massive effect on all areas of your life? In fact, you could say that all things SANE are just tools that help you replace setpoint-elevating habits with setpoint-lowering habits as easily, enjoyably, and sustainably as possible.

Now you might be thinking that it is hard to change habits, and you are right. But if we look at the science behind your habits to learn a few tricks, you can make habit change much easier.

Every day, your brain must complete millions of complex tasks. Whether you're brushing your teeth or driving to work, your brain creates habits so you don't have to think about each and every thing you do during the day. Otherwise, you would quickly become overwhelmed and never be able to successfully navigate your busy life.

Consider driving your car. When you first were learning to drive, you had to make sure the mirrors were in the correct place, your seat belt was buckled, the engine was on, the parking brake was off, the lights were on, and so on. Then you put your car into gear and carefully backed out of your garage and checked for oncoming traffic. Next, you looked at each street sign to make sure you were making the correct turns. Before it became habitual, driving took 100 percent of your attention.

Now, it's likely driving has become so habitual that it happens almost automatically. Have you ever driven somewhere and then for just a second thought to yourself, "How did I get here?" Your habits were in the driver's seat, while you were thinking about something else. That's the magic of habits, but it is also the reason that setpoint-elevating habits can become so hard to overcome. It's like they are driving your actions, and therefore driving your setpoint up. At least until now! Here's how we'll get you back in the driver's seat.

THE HABIT LOOP

To learn how you can easily create new setpoint-lowering habits, you first need to understand what researchers call the "habit loop"—a continuous cycle of *cue*, *routine*, and *reward* that underlies all habitual behavior. First, the cue is what sets the entire habit in motion. It could be the time of day, an emotion that makes you reach for your favorite snack, or some other triggering event or place. The cue basically tells your brain: "Okay, you don't have to think anymore. You can go into automatic mode now."

Second, the routine is what makes up the core of the habit. This refers to the action, thought, or feeling triggered by the cue, and it either moves you further away from your goals or brings you closer to them. In the case of mindlessly snacking on the couch (a routine) during your favorite show (a cue), or hitting the fast-food drive-through (a routine) after work (a cue), such actions can have a negative impact on your setpoint.

The third part of habit and the part that makes habits almost like an addiction is the reward. This is what creates the feeling of anticipation and even cravings that accompany a lot of your habits. Whatever the reward is, it trains your brain, using feel-good chemicals such as serotonin and dopamine to search out the cue and perform the behavior so that you can then experience the reward of these feel-good chemicals. The reward can be almost anything. It can be the comfort you feel from eating a big bowl of ice cream. It can be the satisfying salty crunch of potato chips after a long day. On the other hand, it can also be the calm energy you feel after enjoying a SANE workout or smoothie.

The important thing to remember is that every time you get into a habit loop, your actions, emotions, and feelings become more and more intertwined and interconnected until the process becomes nearly automatic, without any conscious effort on your part—for better or worse. But when you understand how a habit works, you can change habits and take back control of your life without any willpower or calorie counting.

THE EASIEST WAY TO CHANGE A SETPOINT-ELEVATING HABIT

Once a habit has been formed—such as eating a sugary snack every afternoon—the cue and the reward are always in your brain. The cue-and-reward portion of a habit are the hardest to change because, as we talked about, it is hard for your brain *not* to do something. Try telling your brain not to be triggered when three o'clock rolls around and sugary snacks start calling your name. Try telling your brain not to feel happy and rewarded as you bite into that candy bar. Even though you know this habit isn't doing your setpoint any favors, you can't "try harder" *not* to feel the cue and the reward. However, the middle part of your habit loop—the routine—is the easiest part to change because it is based on *doing*, and your brain loves doing things.

To overcome harmful habits, it is essential to identify the cues and underlying rewards that drive your habitual behavior so that you can see the habit loop in action. This can require a great deal of self-examination and quiet reflection, especially for those habits that are deeply ingrained in your brain. But once you become aware of specific habit triggers and understand the desired rewards, you can interrupt the cycle and insert new, helpful routines to close the habit loops. In fact, it's fine to use the same cue and same reward and simply replace the routine in a habit you already have.

As an example, let's take snacking on potato chips in the evening while watching TV. The cue is turning on the TV. You just automatically reach for something crunchy on your way to the couch. It's not even a conscious decision anymore.

Now what is the reward in this case? There are probably two. One is that you get to relieve tension from a long day while spending time with your favorite TV programs. There is also the crunchy, salty taste of potato chips. In this case, you don't need to replace your TV watching because it provides relaxation—which we all need. However, it would be helpful to find a replacement routine or a setpoint-lowering substitution for the chips. My suggestion would be to replace the potato chips with a snack that is SANE but also provides the salty crunch, such as kale chips or baked pork rinds.

So the cue (watching TV) and the reward (relaxation along with a scrumptious salty, crunchy snack) stay exactly the same. All you did was replace one small part of the routine with a SANE alternative. Remember, you never want to focus on what you want to avoid, but rather focus on what you want to *do*. You want to fill your life—and in this case your habit loops—with so much SANE goodness that you automatically crowd out the inSANEity.

SANE Habit Upgrades: Getting Started

In the previous chapter, you learned an effective way to start creating new habits using intention implementations. Also, by swapping sugary juice for a SANE smoothie, for example, you discovered how to take an unhealthy habit and easily transform it into a healthy one. Seeing how manageable and empowering this is, you may be thinking already about the many small habits in your life where you could easily replace a negative routine with a positive routine. Well, let's make it official and write down five setpoint-elevating habits that you could work on upgrading. These could involve eating inSANE foods or shaming yourself.

Go ahead and write down those five habits now.

Look at the list you just created and identify one of the unhelpful habits that you would like to replace with a helpful habit. Write down the cue, the routine, and the reward you get from that habit. Then write down three possible replacements—SANE substitutions—for the routine. If the habit involves food, use the SANE substitution charts in Chapter 8 to help you replace setpoint-elevating routines with setpoint-lowering routines.

Circle one of the three substitutions that seems the most doable. Take a moment to look at what you circled, and make a promise to yourself that you will work on this new SANE substitution routine for a week and then see how you feel. If it doesn't work, that's just part of the learning process. All it means is that your substitution is not satisfying the reward piece of the habit. Don't let shame and discouragement sneak in. Try a different substitution and practice it until you get it right. Starting small will help you to build serious momentum in changing other habits.

Every one of your habits either raises or lowers your setpoint, and like your setpoint, they can be changed. But please don't try to erase or break a bad habit. Remember, attacking the negative works *against* your brain and therefore isn't effective. Instead, pursue the positive and *do* something (rather than not doing something), and replace a setpoint-elevating behavior with a new setpoint-lowering behavior. Stack a few of these SANE habit upgrades on top of each other and your habits will lower your setpoint for you while you focus on enjoying your new naturally slim life.

FOOD AS A FIX

When it comes to putting things into your body, inSANE eating habits can become full-on addictions with life-threatening consequences. But at what point do habits turn into addictions?

To answer that question, it helps to understand the difference between a habit and an addiction. In simplest terms, the primary difference between the two is that you are ultimately in control of a habit, while an addiction is in control of you. Or consider my father's take on it (he's a chemical addiction counselor):

"Non-addicts use habits to feel good. Addicts use their habits not to feel bad." For example, if you enjoy a cup of coffee in the morning and could function fine without it, you have a habit. However, if you feel terrible and cannot function unless you drink a cup of coffee, you may be addicted to caffeine.

While food addiction has not been officially recognized by the *DSM-V* (the current edition of the *Diagnostic and Statistical Manual of Mental Disorders* used by mental health professionals), it has updated the diagnostics for binge eating disorder (BED) to suggest that future editions will officially recognize food addiction as a substance addiction.

If you have ever found yourself compelled to overeat, eating compulsively, or regularly bingeing on a specific food, even when you don't want to (and you know it's going to make you feel horrible), you may have fallen victim to a food addiction.

Symptoms of Food Addiction

Looking over the following symptoms, have you ever experienced any of these in conjunction with your eating habits?

- Eating certain foods when not hungry or at odd times of the day.
- Worrying and thinking obsessively about cutting back on certain foods.
- Feeling tired and sluggish after eating problem foods instead of energized and alive.
- Experiencing cravings or obsessively thinking about certain types of foods.
- Mindlessly continuing to eat large amounts of certain foods, even though they are no longer enjoyable, even when you realize the consequences.
- Developing an increased tolerance for food in which you need more to achieve the same effect.
- Experiencing withdrawal that has a significant negative impact if you stop.

- Losing control over how much you eat of problem foods and when to stop eating them.
- Allowing food and eating to interfere with important activities of life.
- Ignoring the negative consequences of a food addiction.

Perhaps you never thought of food as being addictive. But when you consider that possibility, it can explain why conventional "just try harder" dieting can't work for you.

One of the hallmarks of addiction is the inability to stop once you have had just a little—just one drink or one bite. That is why if you do identify with a food addiction, anyone telling you "everything in moderation" needs to stop misleading you. It's not helpful to tell an alcoholic "everything in moderation," and if your brain is addicted to a certain food, nobody should give you the same harmful advice.

But this can be good news, because it means if food addiction is a problem for you, there is a simple solution. Researchers have found that certain types of foods act in the same way on your brain as alcohol or drugs. A 2002 study analyzed more than 100 peer-reviewed articles, each of which showed that humans produce opioids—the active ingredient in heroin and other narcotics—after digesting excessive sugars and fats (Kelley et al. 2002). They went on to discover that our brain chemicals can cause physical cravings for these foods and act as a significant and frequent trigger of bingeing behavior.

There's more: In 2009, researchers from Yale University created the Food Addiction Scale, a 25-point questionnaire to assess food addiction in individuals (Gearhardt et al. 2009). Over the years, it has been used in study after study to confirm that people can become addicted to certain processed foods, such as bread. This is new and important information that starvation diet programs ignore. And that's heartbreaking because, again, telling someone who is addicted to a processed food like bread to "just eat smaller portions" is as reasonable and effective as telling someone who is addicted to nicotine to "just smoke shorter cigarettes."

Let's say that your diet focuses on reducing the quantity of what you eat (versus the quality of what you eat). This means that you are encouraged to eat small portions of the food you are addicted to—for instance, bread. So you do what you are told, and you eat the food. Then the reward and addiction chemicals and circuitry in your brain kick in, and your cravings for that forbidden food become even *stronger*.

Moderation doesn't pour water on the flames of addiction; it pours gasoline on them. Trying to diet that way can, at best, leave you feeling constantly deprived and depleted and, at worst, can *cause* diabetes, obesity, heart disease, cancer, and Alzheimer's, because it *causes* you to eat more of the addictive processed foods that can lead to these devastating diseases.

Scientists have found that the most addictive "foods" are sugar, fat, flour, wheat, salt, artificial sweeteners, and caffeine. So, it is no surprise that the most highly addictive products are processed foods that combine these addictive ingredients into a deadly mix, such as bread, doughnuts, French fries, snack foods, cookies, fast food, candy, pasta, and chips.

Just knowing that some foods are addictive, however, doesn't necessarily help you overcome addiction. Let's be very clear—overcoming an addiction is one of life's biggest challenges. But here's the key: We have NO chance of overcoming an addiction with strategies that encourage us to consume—but in smaller portions—the addictive substance. The fact is that you CAN break free from food addiction and emotional eating. But this different result requires a different approach. Getting where you want to go isn't about monitoring points, calories, or portions even closer. But if you focus on eating so much delicious SANE food that you are too full for addictive and toxic processed foods, your lowered setpoint will "pull" you to your goal weight and optimal health—and more importantly—keep you there effortlessly.

The SANE Solution to Food Addiction and Emotional Eating

To start breaking free from inSANE food addiction, create an inventory of what foods cause you the most trouble. Write these foods down in your journal or notebook. Look over your list. Circle the top three foods that you think you might be addicted to, or that at the very least cause you to eat more than you want to.

Next to each of those foods, write down some of the feelings that you associate with them—for example, shame, loneliness, guilt, pleasure, anger, sadness, abandonment, and pride, to name just a few. There is no right or wrong answer, and no judgment.

Then select one food on your list and promise to yourself that you will work on freeing yourself from it this week. I'll help you with the "how" in the next section, but for now it is essential to understand how transformative it is to recognize triggering events and your resulting emotions. Awareness is the first step. This improves your ability to choose more helpful reactions to your emotions. It opens the door to finding ways to avoid the trigger or to make a SANE Substitution to help you deal with the trigger. You take back your control. You take back your health. You take back your life!

BUT WHAT ABOUT WILLPOWER?

The conventional dieting "wisdom" that has led to skyrocketing rates of overweight, depression, anxiety, eating disorders, body shame, and diabetes tells you that willpower is the number-one key to your success. But it is a scientific fact that willpower cannot lead to *enjoyable and lasting* weight loss. Period. The definition of willpower is the ability to force yourself to do something you do not enjoy. That isn't sustainable.

This doesn't mean that willpower is bad or that zero willpower is required to lower your setpoint SANEly. However, it does mean that any plan promising *enjoyable and lasting* weight loss must do two things:

1. Require *less* willpower over time (not more).
2. Help you develop *more* willpower (not diminish your existing willpower).

The first one is simple, so let's cover that first. The longer you starve yourself, the more willpower it requires to starve yourself. You can eat 1,200 calories today without too much willpower. However, 1 week from now it will require way more willpower, and 1 month from now it will require so much willpower that more than 90 percent of people will rightly conclude "it's not worth it!"

Compare that to eating more non-starchy vegetables like broccoli. Eating more broccoli may require a bit of willpower today. Do it daily and a week from today it will require less willpower. Keep doing it daily and a month from now it will require "negative" willpower. That is, you will have acquired a taste for broccoli and enjoy eating it. This means that while "eat less" requires more and more willpower over time and therefore harms you, "eat more, SANEly" requires less and less willpower over time and therefore heals you.

HOW TO DEVELOP MORE WILLPOWER

I've got some encouraging news for you: Willpower can be developed and strengthened just like a muscle. I've also got a groundbreaking tip for you: Focus your willpower on developing willpower. Think of it like the old riddle where a genie says you can have three wishes and you wish for more wishes. Starvation dieting wastes wishes. SANE living leverages your wishes (willpower) to get you more wishes (willpower)!

Here's how this works: An area of your brain called the *prefrontal cortex* affects willpower. It controls learning, memory, and decision-making, and it's highly connected to other brain regions, such as those involved with addictions and rewards. Specifically, the cells in the middle of your prefrontal cortex help you say yes to your goals and no to your temptations. The faster these brain cells "fire," or transmit messages to other brain cells, the better you are at resisting temptation. If these brain cells become inflamed, they will not fire as quickly, and your willpower goes down.

Exerting willpower forces your brain to expend a lot of energy in the form of glucose, which it may not have if you are hungry or unable to metabolize glucose as efficiently due to poor sleep or stress. Starvation and stress wreak havoc in the prefrontal cortex. It's as if you have brain damage in areas in which you need self-control. The net effect is that the starvation and shame-based approach to weight loss *causes* you to have less willpower. This is why people on diets often feel like people who are trying to give up smoking: on edge, easily annoyed, snapping at loved ones, and more.

Really let that sink in. Conventional starvation and shame programs encourage you to stress and will your way to starving yourself. But starvation and stress reduce your willpower. That's like having a power outage, and your power company telling you to turn on your TV to watch for updates. They are telling you to use your willpower to do things that compromise your very ability to use willpower.

A SANEr approach is to tap into the science of heart rate variability (HRV), or the beat-to-beat fluctuations in heart rate. In addition to your brain, your heart plays a key role in willpower. In a 2007 study published in *Psychological Science*, researchers asked participants to flex their willpower by eating carrots and resisting cookies (Segerstrom and Nes 2007). When they successfully ate carrots and resisted cookies, their HRV was elevated. When participants had a drop in HRV, the opposite happened: They ate cookies and resisted carrots. High HRV = high willpower. Low HRV = low willpower.

This is great because by understanding what impacts HRV, you can upgrade it and therefore develop more willpower (instead of diminishing it through starvation dieting and calorie counting). Changes in HRV are determined by the two parts of your nervous system, your sympathetic nervous system (when you are alert) and your parasympathetic nervous system (when you are calm).

When you are anxious, stressed out, tired, or starving, your sympathetic nervous system takes over. This is the branch of your nervous system responsible for your "fight or flight" mechanism. It helps your body to respond quickly to perceived threats or stress. When this happens, your heart rate goes up but HRV goes down.

But when you are feeling calm and relaxed, your parasympathetic nervous system is in control. You will experience a lower heart rate but HRV goes up. You are then able to effortlessly manage stress, control impulsive behavior, and flex your willpower, although it won't seem like you are trying. It's like how everything seems to require less effort when you are in a "good place." Imagine if you were always in that "good place." That's what we're after. Swimming *with* the current of your body, heart, and brain, rather than against it.

So in a real-life example: If you are in a "bad place"—that is, you are anxious, stressed, and tired because you are starving—when you see a box of free doughnuts, your heart rate increases, but HVR decreases. You have less willpower. In other words, you have been using willpower to starve yourself, which reduces your willpower both in that moment and your baseline willpower reserves. Therefore, when you see the doughnuts, you don't have enough willpower to pass them by. In sum: Starvation dieting causes the very thing you are trying to avoid.

However, if you are in a "good place"—that is, full and satisfied by an abundance of SANE setpoint-lowering foods—when you see a box of doughnuts, your heart rate decreases, but your HRV increases. You have more willpower. In fact, you have so much willpower that you walk by the box of doughnuts without a second thought.

Here's how to make that happen in your life:

The SANE Solution to Develop More Willpower

Going back to our genie metaphor, if you want "infinite willpower wishes," all you need to do is focus your willpower on increasing your HRV. Again, the only thing I want you using your willpower for is getting even more willpower. Here's how you do that:

1. Use a bit of willpower to eat so much setpoint-lowering SANE food that you are too full for inSANE food.
2. Use a bit of willpower to do less, but exercise smarter.
3. Use a bit of willpower to find ways to sleep more.

Each of these increases HRV and therefore your willpower while in and of themselves requiring less willpower over time. How cool is that? For decades you were told to use your willpower to starve yourself, which not only sapped your willpower but also required more and more willpower over time. Now you are investing a small bit of willpower in developing more willpower and will need less and have even more over time.

If you want even more willpower, I've got two more tools for you: SANE breathing and meditation techniques. Studies have shown HRV starts increasing as your breathing rate drops below 12 breaths per minute. You can try this yourself. Breathe in and out slowly. Each breath should take 10 to 15 seconds. Focus on exhaling more slowly. For best results, you slow down breathing to 4 to 6 breaths per minute. That's 10 to 15 seconds per breath.

In addition to breathing exercises, specific types of meditation can increase the amount of gray matter in your prefrontal cortex, thus boosting your HRV and thus boosting your willpower, thus making a lower setpoint even easier. On the 21-Day Plan in Chapter 15, you will find a quick type of meditation that will not only help you love yourself more, but also relax you so that your HRV increases.

SUPPORT AND GRATITUDE

The two remaining SANE mind-set tools are important to lowering your setpoint: a loving community and gratitude.

A Loving Community

A loving community involves participating in the *right kind* of support group. "Right kind" is important because conventional starvation and shame-based support groups help you lower your setpoint as much as getting together with drinking buddies at a bar helps you quit drinking. They don't. But assuming you are in a support group focused on love and science instead of shame and starvation, happy days are soon to follow. For example, a study from the *European Journal of Clinical Nutrition* reported that "social support is important to achieve beneficial changes in risk factors for disease, such as overweight and obesity" (Verheijden et al. 2005).

Another study published in the *International Journal of Medicine* showed that online support groups specifically were especially effective at allowing participants to reach their goal weight and to maintain that weight longer than those who did not have the benefit of support (Hwang et al. 2011). Besides increasing the overall level of participants' weight loss, the study also found three other key areas in which online support communities provided tangible benefits for the members.

First, online support groups offer encouragement and motivation that is hard to find outside of a structured program. Individuals report that being part of a family-like online community is a great way to receive encouragement and motivation to stick with changes that can be hard to stick with when you are alone. The support of like-minded individuals also allowed members to recover from mistakes and overcome barriers more easily.

Also, while we all get frustrated with technology sometimes, being able to get loving support and help anytime and anywhere—rather than just once a week after spending an hour driving to a meeting—is a big benefit of being part of a loving online community.

Second, another key area the study explored was that sharing experiences was critical in many members' finding success. Members who discussed and shared common goals, struggles, and experiences found it easier to stick with their plans. Consistent sharing with other members combats loneliness and isolation, helps with accountability, and makes people feel like they were part of something bigger and more meaningful.

Now before we go too far, again, you don't just need support; you need the *right* form of support. In fact, if you've tried "support groups" in the past and they let you down, it's not because support groups are bad or that you are bad, but perhaps the support group you tried wasn't right for you.

The good news is that will never happen again because you are about to discover how to pick the perfect form of support to meet your unique needs and challenges. You want to find a group that is curated by a loving, caring, scientifically accurate, and professionally trained coaching staff.

Also, be wary of "calorie counting" and "pounds lost" focused groups. The point of an effective group is not to compete or show off. Remember process goals versus results goals from the previous chapter. Your ideal support system is about motivation, accountability, and encouragement to reach your personal goals. If you feel bad because you aren't as "good" as someone else, or because a "better" member lost half a pound more than you for the week, find a different support group.

Helpful Support Group	Harmful Support Group
Professionally moderated and scientifically modern (uses up-to-date methods)	Random people on the Internet
Only loving, caring members focused on making progress	Negative members focused on shortcomings and looking for someone to blame for their problems
Cooperative	Competitive
Peer support	The "perfect" versus the "imperfect"
Safe and secure	Members attacking other members or passing judgment on shortcomings
Honest and open	Guarded, walking on eggshells, scared of saying the wrong thing
Clear focus on shared purpose	Confusing, misleading information and invalidating debates
Loving acceptance	Full of "shoulds"
Consistent sharing	A feeling of randomness and inconsistency

Tip: If you are interested in participating in the premium support group at SANESolution.com, email your receipt for this book to Service@SANESolution.com to get a reader-only discount.

The SANE Solution to Getting Setpoint-Lowering Support

As you may have heard in high school and college: Get involved! In a large study, researchers looked at about 5,400 people who participated in an online support program for at least 6 months and who posted at least twice during the study period in the online forum. The researchers found the most significant factor that increased a participant's weight loss was a person's level of engagement within the online group. After 6 months, individuals who were most deeply involved lost more than twice as much weight as those who were least involved in the online support group. That's a dramatic increase in weight loss and the only difference was the level of love and support they got and gave in a SANE online support group! No starvation. No endless hours at the gym. They literally loved their way to weight loss!

So the moral of the story is pretty simple: If you are serious about losing weight long-term, I highly recommend you immediately get serious about finding a program with a strong online community of genuinely loving and scientifically qualified members and coaches. We do have one at SANESolution.com if you'd like to check it out.

Thank Your Way to a Lower Setpoint

The second part of the almost magical psychological setpoint-lowering equation is the practice of gratitude. Every day. Even if sometimes it might be hard to feel grateful. Here's why: Two psychologists, Dr. Robert A. Emmons of the University of California, Davis, and Dr. Michael E. McCullough of the University of Miami, have conducted extensive research on gratitude. In one study, they asked one group of people to write about things they were grateful for that had occurred during the week, a second group to write about daily irritations or things that had displeased them, and a third to write about events that had affected them (with no emphasis on them being positive or negative) (McCullough et al. 2002).

After 10 weeks, the participants who expressed gratitude in their writings were more optimistic and felt better about their lives. Even better, they also worked out more and had fewer visits to doctors than those who focused on sources of aggravation.

Studies have also shown that people who practice gratitude have 10 percent fewer stress-related illnesses, are more physically fit, and have 12 percent lower blood pressure. They have stronger relationships, are better liked by others, and have stronger community ties. They even make up to 20 percent more per hour and their incomes are roughly 7 percent higher than the average. And finally, practicing being grateful can add up to 7 years to your life!

With all those benefits let me ask you: Have you been grateful or thankful today? If so, that's great! If not, no worries because here's how to get started.

The SANE Solution to Practicing Gratitude

To start, let's tie this back to the critical elements of support and community and pick five people whom you are grateful for right now. They can be family, friends, or maybe someone you haven't seen in a while, or a deceased relative. Heck, it can even be someone you don't know personally, such as a favorite author or musician. Write them down and draw a little smiley face next to them. You can also download and print free reader-only worksheets to help with this at SANESolution.com.

Next, write down five positive things about your health and body. These can be as simple as: "I am grateful for my 20/20 vision," or more specific such as "I love how my eyes light up when I smile." Think about all aspects of your health and body—not just what glossy magazines and daytime TV tell you to focus on. Only by loving who you are can you become who you want to be. Love and caring always beat shame and guilt.

Next, write down five things you have done in the last week that made you proud of yourself. This can be anything from the smallest gesture of kindness to a stranger, such as holding the door for someone, or something that you did to show love to yourself . . . such as taking a 10-minute walk to enjoy the sun.

Next, write down the best part of your day so far. It could be your hot cup of coffee or tea, that cute little bird you saw outside of your window, or even opening your heart and mind for this exercise.

For some people, writing out what they are thankful for is second nature and comes easily. For others, it can feel like a struggle. No matter where you are with your gratitude skills, I want you to promise yourself that you will create a new 3-minute habit of writing down at least three things you are grateful for every day. And please remember, these don't need to be big things. Here are some helpful prompts you may want to use:

What have you done to take care of yourself today?

Was there a beautiful part of nature you saw today?

What put a smile on your face today?

Before we bring this chapter to a close, can we get real for a second? Think back over everything we've covered. How much different is what we've been covering when you compare it to: "Damn it! Just try harder to eat less and stop being so lazy!" Seriously.

It's almost like this SANE setpoint-lowering approach is the exact opposite of the starvation, shame, and stress approach that has beaten you down for decades. And isn't that awesome? After all, if what you did in the past made things worse, doesn't it make sense that something completely different is what we need to make things better?

You are taking a whole new approach and will get a whole new result. You have so much to look forward to. And if nothing else, today's gratitude journal seems like it could be a robust one! Thanks for reading this far. We both have a lot to be grateful for.

SANE Points

- The most powerful way to create change easily and almost effortlessly is to practice awareness and use SANE substitutions to replace negative routines with positive routines. This process reinforces itself and has a huge impact on your health, your setpoint weight, and the quality of your life.
- To break free from addictive emotional eating, understand what triggers the behavior and its resulting emotions. This better empowers you the next time with radically more awareness. Each week select one addicting food and promise to yourself that you will work on freeing yourself from using the tools in this program.
- If you can engage in activities that increase your heart rate variability, you can build your willpower reserve and effortlessly gain control over your behavior. The best use of willpower is to develop more willpower.
- Get involved in a loving support group. This action has enormous value in helping to create lasting change.
- Keep a gratitude journal. Focusing on the good things in your life can lower stress, improve your weight and health, and lead to greater self-compassion and self-love.

CHAPTER 15

The 21-Day SANE Setpoint Solution

If you have reached this chapter after reading all the preceding chapters, please email me at Service@SANESoution.com because I would like to congratulate you. Thank you for being the change we both want to see in the world. You are proving that it is possible to rewrite your story, and from this moment on you will start living the life of your dreams. You are now equipped with the information, motivation, and mind-set required to get everything you deserve out of the therapeutic setpoint-lowering plan you'll find in the following pages. I know you are committed to breaking free from the quick-fix starvation-based "just tell me what to do" approaches that have failed you in the past. You have my guarantee that correct information plus motivation plus SANE mind-set plus proven science and practical engineering will work, always. But you didn't need me to tell you that, did you? After all, you have learned so much about yourself and the science over these past 14 chapters. Well done!

If you have skipped to this chapter, take a moment to ask yourself if the approach of "just tell me what to do" worked in the past. Your future is worth much more than the few hours it will take to read the preceding chapters, and I guarantee that the plan will work radically better after you do. Your life and your ability to fully contribute to the lives of those you love is too important to shortchange yourself. Please only start this plan after reading the preceding chapters. You are worth it. I promise.

As we go through this therapeutic plan together, all I ask is that you give this your *all* for 21 days, and let the inevitable results speak for themselves. Treat the next 21 days with the same sanctity you would if you just had major surgery and need 3 weeks to heal. You and I are here to heal your metabolism, lower your setpoint, and protect you from being another victim of the diabesity epidemic. For just 21 days, nothing is more important than your healing…nothing! You have suffered for too long.

I really need you to give yourself permission to take on this medical recovery mind-set. For the next 21 days, promise me that you will put your physical and emotional health first because…

1. Living your best life isn't unreasonable.
2. You deserve 100 percent of what life has to offer.
3. You cannot afford to live in fear.

REASON #1: LIVING YOUR BEST LIFE ISN'T UNREASONABLE

If you share this 21-Day Plan with someone who hasn't walked the path we just walked together in the previous chapters, they'll likely see it as just another diet, and much of it will seem unreasonable and ridiculous. Living your best life isn't unreasonable. Taking action that improves your ability to enrich the lives of others isn't ridiculous. If improving your quality of life is unreasonable, then maybe getting unreasonable is not a bad thing. Because you see the next 21 days for what they really are—a therapeutic protocol to help you recover from medical issues that have burdened you for decades—everything you are about to read and do will occur to you as not only reasonable, but also essential. For example, if you've ever had surgery, given birth, or lived with someone who did, you know that when a life is on the line, all sorts of otherwise "absurd" lifestyle changes get done almost automatically. Here's the trick: Your life IS on the line. And your life IS worth it. When that message sinks in, everything you'll do over the next 21 days will be a blessing (not a burden).

REASON #2: YOU DESERVE 100 PERCENT OF WHAT LIFE HAS TO OFFER

I'm basically begging you to give this your ALL because you deserve 100 percent of what life has to offer, and for some things in life, putting 90 percent in gives you far less than 90 percent out. For example, if you are 90 percent faithful to your spouse, you will likely not get even close to 90 percent of the benefits of marriage. Similarly, when it comes to treating life-threatening medical issues, being 90 percent faithful to your recovery will not get you 90 percent of the benefits.

This therapeutic plan is only 3 weeks, and I know that you can give 100 percent for 3 weeks. Look at you. Look at all the challenges you have overcome in your life. You've done so much more than what I'll ask of you. Remember how capable, courageous, competent, and committed you are, and give 100 percent of yourself to these next 21 days. I promise that your experience of life and of yourself will transform forever.

Remember, the key that changes everything about weight loss and wellness with this plan is that you and I are operating in the SANE world of science and engineering—not the insane world of anecdotes and gimmicks. This means you never need to take anyone else's "word for it" ever again. Eat, move, and live the way we're discussing, and your setpoint will fall. Always. For everyone. It's proven science combined with practical engineering.

This therapeutic setpoint-lowering plan will transform and ultimately save your life, while forever freeing you from all the confusing and conflicting weight-loss information that has failed you in the past. Imagine a life in which you feel attractive and healthy, proud of who you are, excited about your life, treated with respect by others, truly living. You deserve all of that and so much more. In just 21 days you will not only realize your worth, but you will also live it, 100 percent of the time. Not because I say so. But because modern science proves it. Because practical engineering enables it. And again, because you are worth it.

During these 21 days, you'll jump-start an enjoyable, sustainable, and simple way of living that will unlock that naturally thin person within you. Once you have completed the plan, you will have graduated into "living SANE," fully empowered to continue a way of life that finally gives you what you've longed for in terms of leanness, better health, and self-worth. #SANE4Life

The only "catch" is that I DO need you to let go of the past and give yourself *completely* to 3 weeks that will *completely* change your future. But don't worry, here's a simple mind-set shift that makes this so much easier.

REASON #3: YOU CANNOT AFFORD TO LIVE IN FEAR

Please don't let temporary fear of unfamiliar methods keep you trapped within that old familiar pain of an elevated setpoint. You see, the new foods, exercises, and habits in your 21-Day Plan may not seem easy at first, but honestly not because they are hard. Rather, they may *seem* hard at first just because they are not familiar. I bet you have experienced this in your life before. For instance, have you ever been in a new area and struggled to get to the grocery store or bank? Was that because going to the grocery store or bank is hard? No. It's because you were doing something easy in an unfamiliar place. That's what this is.

Eating a lot more of specific setpoint-lowering foods, moving your body for a few minutes in a new way, and sleeping a lot more (the three primary keys to this plan) are easy. You've done things much harder than each of them for decades. However, you will now be doing them in a new place: in the land of SANEity instead of the familiar but toxic land of starvation, shame, and stress. You will never be hungry. You will never feel deprived. You will never need to spend hours exercising. You will not need to skimp on sleep. You will be SANE. And that *will* be unfamiliar, but it *will not* be hard for someone like you. And it *will* work if you let it.

You are about to discover the possibility of eating quality food, exercising smartly, and never obsessing over calories or worrying about willpower or shame again. You will begin to feel more alive than you can imagine—physically, mentally, and emotionally. Your clothes will get looser. You will have more energy. You will think more clearly. You will make love more passionately. You will see yourself as valuable and worthy again. You will feel great about yourself—no more blue moods, no more self-conscious worry about going out in public, no more negative ideas about yourself. You will be excited about life again. Everything you want out of life is on the other side of eating the most nutritious food, doing the most healing exercise, adopting a SANE mind-set, and resting. Thank you for letting me be your coach. This is going to be incredible.

THE 21-DAY THERAPEUTIC SETPOINT-LOWERING PLAN

To guarantee you a SANE life and the transformative results of a lower setpoint, this plan gives you the most potent and powerful week-by-week packaging of SANE nutrition, activity, nutraceuticals, lifestyle habits, and psychology ever created. You will get access to every single tool necessary to get you to your lower setpoint and optimum weight as quickly, safely, and easily as possible. If instead you are looking for a way to ease into lowering your setpoint, or to maintain a lower setpoint simply, please jump ahead to the next chapter. However, if you want to lower your setpoint as much as possible in the next 21 days, get ready to transform, and get ready to give all of yourself to healing all of yourself.

The plan is set up in a 3-week format, with a sample day representing each week. That sample day gives you an easy-to-follow, nearly hour-by-hour SANE routine that can be adapted to your schedule and tastes and replicated accordingly over 7 days. A positive, consistent routine you stick to—waking up at the same time, eating your meals at the same time, and doing other activities at the same time—sets you up for success. Remember the power of habits. When you do the same setpoint-lowering things every day, living SANEly becomes second nature, and no willpower is needed.

Day by day, you'll progress toward a lower setpoint with SANE eating guidelines—without counting calories or obsessing over every little morsel that passes through your lips. You'll do SANE physical activities that will re-engineer the way your body works and looks. Far from starving, you will be strong…in every sense of the word. And every day, you will work on your attitude and mindset so that you'll start feeling great about yourself and optimistic about what you're accomplishing.

Over the next 3 weeks, this plan will reprogram your body to lower your setpoint by 10 pounds in 21 days. Yes, your body will fight for you to be 10 pounds lighter, forever. If you follow this plan, it doesn't matter who you are or what you've done in the past—you will get results. Every element of this plan was specifically engineered to heal your body and dramatically lower your setpoint.

Now is the time to go for it, because there is nothing that can hold you back. But before you begin the 21 days, here are some simple reminders and guidelines so that you get focused and excited about what is going to happen. Also, know that you have an entire team, a loving community, and a complimentary personalized program available to you at SANESolution.com.

GENERAL GUIDELINES

SANE Nutrition

Meal frequency and duration: Eat five meals a day evenly spaced out—for two reasons: First, trying to eat as many non-starchy vegetables as you need to lower your setpoint in fewer than five meals will cause digestive upset. Second, it maximizes muscle protein synthesis (MPS), which will help lower your setpoint. Because you will be sleeping for 8 hours a night, that leaves 16 hours to eat 5 meals, so you should be eating approximately every 3 hours.

The slower you eat, the lower your setpoint. Ideally, you will take no less than 20 minutes to eat your *complete* SANE meals (non-starchy vegetables and nutrient-dense protein). This doesn't mean you need to sit at a table and eat for 20 minutes. That 20 minutes can include time in your car, eating at your desk, and so on. The goal is simply to avoid "wolfing" down food in just a couple of minutes.

Every meal contains:

3 to 4 servings optimal non-starchy veggies (ONSV)
1 serving of 25 to 50 grams optimal nutrient-dense protein (ONDP)
   (2 servings per day must come from an optimal source)

Optimal Non-Starchy Veggies (ONSV)

Alfalfa, arugula, bok choy, barley grass, Brussels sprouts, chard, garlic, greens, kale, kelp, mixed greens, moringa, neem, romaine lettuce, seaweed, spinach, spirulina, watercress, wheat grass, asparagus, broccoli, red cabbage, mushrooms, onions, and artichokes

Serving size information can be found in Chapter 15.

Optimal Nutrient-Dense Protein (ONDP) and Nutrient-Dense Protein (NDP)

Two daily servings of 25 to 50 grams from any of these optimal sources: salmon, tuna, oysters, clams, mussels, sardines, anchovies, sea bass, or organ meats

Remaining NDP may come from: clean grass-fed whey protein concentrate, grass-fed beef, very lean conventional beef, turkey, white meat chicken, or seafood

Serving size information can be found in Chapter 15.

Every day contains:

Optimal Whole-Food Fats

One serving from the following sources: coconut, undutched cocoa/cacao, avocado, flax seeds, chia seeds, macadamia nuts, olives, coconut flour, cocoa/cacao nibs, eggs

Serving size information can be found in Chapter 15.

As many SANE superfoods as possible:

Raw undutched cocoa/cacao, garlic, ginger, guar gum, lemons, cinnamon, undistilled apple cider vinegar, low-fat and low-sugar fermented foods, clean and no-sugar-added superfood powders

Use the SANE Plate and paint-by-numbers approach to create your meals, smoothies, and SANE Recipes.

A SANE DAY MENU

Here is a *rough* template for what a day's menu could look like. It's simple because when it comes to sustainable weight loss, simple equals practical equals effective. There is more detail below. Please remember that serving sizes are relative to the size of your hand and do not need to be precise. The exact measures given are illustrative only because a lower setpoint makes precise serving sizes unnecessary.

Meal #1

- No less than 5 ounces of ideally ONDP; normal NDP is okay but not…optimal.
- 1 SANE All-Veggie Smoothie
- If ONDP is not seafood, then take 1 teaspoon of cod liver oil or a double dose of fish oil capsules.

Meal #2 (optional)

- 1 SANE Meal Smoothie (NSVs and nutrient-dense protein) OR
- 1 CLEAN high-prebiotic fiber and protein bar + 1 SANE All-Veggie Smoothie

Meal #3

- No less than 5 ounces of ideally ONDP; normal NDP is okay but not…optimal.
- 1 to 2 servings SANE All-Veggie Soup or Smoothie
- If ONDP is not seafood, then take 1 teaspoon of cod liver oil or a double dose of fish oil capsules.

Meal #4 (optional)

- Same as Meal #2

Meal #5

- No less than 5 ounces ONDP—or NDP, if you've had 2 servings of ONDPs.
- 1 to 2 servings SANE Optimal Veggie Soup or Smoothie
- If ONDP is not seafood, then take 1 teaspoon of cod liver oil or a double dose of fish oil capsules.

Note: If you are going to eat protein/meal bars and want to lower your setpoint, they must contain at least 20 grams of high-quality and clean protein, at least 10 grams of prebiotic fiber, no added sugars, no gluten, no soy, and nothing artificial. As of this writing, the only protein and meal bars formulated with the specific nutrients to optimally lower your setpoint are the bars my company makes. Remember, they are not in any way, shape, or form required, so this isn't a sales pitch. However, if you are going to eat bars while on the 21-Day Plan, the only bars that are designed to lower your setpoint are SANE bars.

On the days you exercise smarter (i.e., twice per week): substitute the following for your fifth meal:

- 8-ounce sweet potato (you can season with anything natural and noncaloric such as salt or cinnamon, but no butter or oil)
- 1 to 2 servings SANE Optimal Veggie Soup or Smoothie
- If you are still hungry, have 4 ounces of additional sweet potato.

During the 21-Day Plan, this substitution helps to prevent cravings and to ensure setpoint lowering versus starvation response in your body. During these 21 days only, the specific form of starch found in sweet potatoes eaten at this specific quantity at this specific time helps to optimize your metabolic rate, thyroid hormone output, sympathetic nervous system activity, appetite hormones, and sex hormones.

SANE Beverages

Drink at least 1 gallon of liquids daily, coming from a combination of any of the following:

- SANE smoothies (1 to 3 daily)
- Water or SANE vitamin water
- Green/white/black tea
- No- or extremely low-sugar kombucha

Tip: Coffee without anything inSANE added to it is fine but doesn't count toward your gallon goal because of its diuretic effects.

SANE Nutraceuticals

Each day, if you choose to take nutraceuticals, include some or all of the following in the plan, divided up as evenly as possible across your meals. Don't worry if this isn't possible for some (e.g., liquid D3 caps can't be divided). Just do your best. The only exception is ZMA, which should be taken on an empty stomach with as little water as possible 30 minutes before bed:

> Inositol (1,000 milligrams)
>
> Choline (1,000 milligrams)
>
> Betaine HCl (100 milligrams), B12 (100 micrograms), and
>   biotin (450 micrograms)
>
> Methionine (1,000 milligrams)
>
> L-carnitine (600 to 1,200 milligrams)
>
> Chromium picolinate (200 micrograms)
>
> Coenzyme Q10 (CoQ10) (10 milligrams)
>
> Vitamin D3 (5,000 IU)
>
> Probiotics and prebiotics (as directed on the bottle)
>
> High EPA and DHA fish oil (at least 1 teaspoon cod liver oil or a double
>   dose of fish oil capsules with breakfast, lunch, and dinner; double
>   that if you wish)
>
> L-leucine (2 grams per meal)
>
> L-glutamine (5 grams daily)
>
> ZMA (3 capsules daily for men or 2 capsules daily for women,
>   preferably on an empty stomach, 30 to 60 minutes before bedtime)

SANE Physical Activity

For the first 2 weeks of your first 21-Day Plan, you will ease your way into smarter exercise. Beginning in week 3, you'll begin the full-on smarter exercise we covered in Chapter 15. After your first cycle, your goal is 20 minutes of full-on smarter exercise weekly.

Once you are exercising smarter:

- Do 10 minutes of eccentric exercise session weekly.
- Do 10 minutes of smarter interval training weekly.

- Ensure you wait at least 2 days in between smarter exercise sessions (i.e., don't do eccentrics and intervals on the same day or on back-to-back days).

Every week, do as much restorative activity as possible. Walk, dance, do yoga, stretch, or enjoy anything else that restores and energizes you (i.e., doesn't stress or bore you). Take at least 10,000 steps daily. Try to do 20 minutes of your restorative activity *outside* daily. Sunlight and nature in general have been shown to have positive hormonal and psychological effects.

The SANE Mind-Set

The 21-Day Plan incorporates various activities that help you achieve your goals, magnify your successes, and become more loving toward yourself. Each day, set aside a few minutes to do a quick meditation, goal-setting exercise, habit change exercise, and gratitude journaling.

Daily Meditation Practice: Each week you will have a different daily meditation to practice. Set aside at least 5 minutes per day for this practice (working your way up to 20 minutes eventually). Set a soft and nonstartling alarm before you begin so that you do not feel distracted or anxious about the time. Practice alone in a quiet place such as your office with the door closed, your bedroom, or even in your parked car.

The setup: Lie down on your back with your palms up. If your low back hurts, bend your knees and put your feet on the floor with your knees resting against each other. If getting down onto the floor is difficult or not feasible, sit comfortably with your feet firmly on the floor and your back and head resting against something so that you can relax and still support the spine. Place your hands palms up wherever is comfortable.

The practice: Close your eyes and softly imagine your upper and lower eyelashes knitting together so it takes no effort to keep your eyes closed. Breathe easily and naturally in through your nose and out through your nose. Allow the body to become heavy, resisting any urge to fidget. If you fidget at first, no worries! Just stay with it. It gets easier with practice, I promise. Once you feel calm and relaxed, begin your practice. If your mind wanders (and it will!) during your practice, gently guide it back to the breath and back to the practice without judgment.

To finish: When you feel complete or when your timer goes off, give yourself a smile, and begin to gently bring small movements into the fingers and toes, then the wrists and feet, gently waking up the body as you slowly open the eyes. If you are on the floor, gently roll to your right side and then use your hands and elbows to sit yourself up.

Other Setpoint-Lowering Tools

- If you are not hungry, and if not eating doesn't cause you to have cravings later in the day, you do not have to eat five meals. However, a minimum of 2 *complete* meals (non-starchy vegetables and nutrient-dense protein) must be eaten daily.
- (Optionally) Mix 2 teaspoons of raw undistilled apple cider vinegar with 8 ounces of water and drink it quickly prior to every meal. This helps with digestion, prevents gas and bloating, and promotes gut healing.
- Get 8 hours of total sleep; one of these can come from naps. Sleep aids are permitted if necessary. It's nearly impossible to heal your hormones without a therapeutic "dose" of sleep. Sleep more to lose more.
- If essential, either or both of the following can be used to help with cravings daily but only if eaten with a *complete* SANE meal:

  1. **Sweet craving**: 1 CLEAN high-prebiotic fiber and SANE Energy Bite
  2. **Salty/crunchy craving**: 1 serving CLEAN high monounsaturated fat baked/microwaved pork rinds

Environmental Considerations

Some researchers are gathering convincing proof that chemical "obesogens," which are found in everyday items such as plastic food-and-beverage containers, food additives, air pollution, and pesticides, *may* cause your body to create more or bigger fat cells, slow your metabolism, increase your appetite, and therefore elevate your setpoint. The jury is still out on the true effect of obesogens on setpoint and metabolism, but until there is a verdict, here are some suggestions for avoiding or limiting your use of these environmental substances:

- Use glass instead of plastic whenever possible.
- Minimize the ingestion of any additives, colorings, or chemicals.

- Minimize the use of chemicals (e.g., cleaning supplies, beauty products, etc.).

WEEK 1—SAMPLE DAY

6:00 a.m.–8:00 a.m.

WAKE UP

No universal wake-up time fits everyone. Again the key is that by the time you get up, you have had 8 hours of sleep.

EAT A SANE BREAKFAST (MEAL #1)

Scramble 2 whole eggs and 6 egg whites (this is an NDP).

Fix a SANE All-Veggie Green Smoothie to enjoy with your breakfast (or, ideally, simply pick up one you batch prepared over the weekend). If you didn't previously batch blend, make three now, enjoy them on the go throughout your day, and add to your non-starchy vegetable (NSV) goals. For information on how to make SANE smoothies, see Chapter 7.

Drink at least 16 ounces of water or green tea with the meal.

TAKE YOUR NUTRACEUTICALS WITH BREAKFAST

If you are using nutraceuticals, take some of them now. (You will be taking them in divided dosages each day—at breakfast, lunch, and dinner—to maximize their absorption.) If your ONDP is not seafood, take 1 teaspoon of pharmaceutical-grade cod liver oil or a double dose of fish oil capsules.

BREW YOUR MORNING GREEN TEA

For greater hydration, brew a lot of green tea in a little water—eight bags at a time in 12 ounces of hot water. Let it sit for a few minutes, add ice, then drink it within the hour. Do this once in the morning and once in the afternoon, and you are good to go.

PRACTICE GRATITUDE

Pick two or three things, big or small, for which you are grateful and write them down in a journal. You will be surprised to find that this activity cancels out most of your anxieties about starting the day. Alternatively, make a list of things for which you are grateful and review it when you get up in the morning and perhaps again in the evening. By spending time each day expressing gratitude for all the blessings in your life, you become a more positive, mindful, and attentive person.

Examples of what to be grateful for: good friends, money in the bank, your parents and children, owning a home or having a roof over your head, your pets, a comfortable bed, a good job and the ability to earn a living, a beautiful day, your education, the kindness of strangers, rainbows and sunsets, the moon and stars, oceans and rivers, hearing and eyesight, favorite hobbies, your talents, and love.

1. Create Your Plan to Overcome Obstacles and Achieve Your Goal

At the beginning of each week, write out your process goals, which you will break down into Action Steps (the initial push that sets progress toward your long-term goal in motion) and Consistency Steps (the momentum that keeps the ball rolling toward your long-term goals). These are the steps you will take this week to move yourself closer to accomplishing your big results goal. Next, put your goals and obstacles into if/when/then plans (implementation intentions) to get you through the week (don't worry, you can always revisit and adjust your process goals during the week). For example:

My Plan for SANE Restorative Activity:

I will set an alarm to wake me up at 6:00 a.m. every day and an alarm to remind me to get ready for bed at 9:30 p.m. every evening (Action Step). When I get up on Monday, Wednesday, and Thursday I will put on my workout clothes and go outside for a 20-minute walk. If I feel like pushing the snooze button on my alarm clock, then the next day I will put my alarm on the other side of the room so I have to get out of bed to turn it off.

My Plan for SANE Snacking:

I will dig my blender and travel mugs out of the back of the cupboard (Action Step) and have a SANE All-Veggie Smoothie each day this week for my midmorning and midafternoon snack (Consistency Step). If I feel stressed out by lack of time during my workweek, then I will prepare batches of SANE smoothies on Monday and Wednesday evening that I can take to work and shake or reblend when I am ready to drink them.

My Plan for SANE Meal Prep/Eating:

I will clear my fridge and pantry of inSANE foods (Action Step) and I will eat a SANE breakfast, lunch, and dinner each day this week (Consistency Step). If I walk into my kitchen and find inSANE foods, then I will throw them away in order to create a supportive environment for my preparation of SANE meals.

Awareness about habits is fantastic, especially if you want to change them and not let them get in the way of your goals. So each day, think of one harmful habit you would like to replace with a helpful one—and a positive routine you can establish to support that helpful habit.

See Chapter 14 for more how-to info.

To work on habit change, formulate positive replacements for the habit and the routine. Write these out in your journal. Here is an example of what to write:

I will replace my negative habit of buying a candy bar from the vending machine at 2:00 p.m. at work with a positive habit. The cue is the time (2:00 p.m.) and the fact that I feel tired and sluggish (emotion). The routine is mindlessly going to the vending machine and buying the candy bar. The reward is the comfort and temporary lift I get from eating the candy bar. I can replace the habit and the routine by fixing a SANE smoothie at 2:00 p.m. when I feel sluggish (new routine), and it will make me feel positive and energized.

To go one step further: If you feel like you are addicted to certain foods, select a food from which you want to free yourself this week. Decide which SANE substitution will help you do that. For example:

> The food I want to free myself from this week is potato chips (or some other salty, crunch snack food). The SANE substitution I can replace it with is kale chips.

9:00 a.m.–11:00 a.m.

HYDRATE

Keep the momentum from your morning SANE smoothie and green tea going with 16 ounces of water. Staying optimally hydrated is a good way to curb cravings, support your metabolism, and flush out toxins that SANE will help your body eliminate.

PLUG INTO YOUR ONLINE SUPPORT GROUP

Studies have proven that participating in the right online support groups daily (even if just for 5 minutes) can nearly double your long-term results. If you have not joined a SANE support group yet, this morning is a good time to do so. If you are already a SANE member, take 5 minutes this morning to access your communications hub and support group so that you can enjoy some amazing benefits. This one simple task helps hold you accountable, and keeps you moving in a positive direction. What's more, if you visit this help center every day, you can stay current on new tips, tools, and tricks to help maximize your results.

HAVE A MIDMORNING SNACK (MEAL #2—OPTIONAL)

Have 1 SANE Meal Smoothie (NSVs and NDP) or 1 CLEAN high-prebiotic fiber and protein bar plus 1 SANE All-Veggie Smoothie. Also, take 1 teaspoon of pharmaceutical-grade cod liver oil.

12:00 p.m.–2:00 p.m.

EAT A SANE LUNCH (MEAL #3)

Pile a baked or grilled 5-ounce chicken breast (NDP) or a cup of tuna (ONDP) atop a large bed of greens. Drizzle with a little olive oil and balsamic vinegar. This lunch is an example of one you can easily pack in the morning in a container to take to work. With your lunch, have 1 to 2 servings of SANE Optimal Veggie Soup or Smoothie.

Drink at least 16 ounces of water or green tea with the meal.

TAKE YOUR NUTRACEUTICALS WITH LUNCH

If you are using nutraceuticals, take some of them now. (You will be taking them in divided dosages each day—at breakfast, lunch, and dinner—to maximize their absorption.) If your ONDP is not seafood, take 1 teaspoon of pharmaceutical-grade cod liver oil or a double dose of fish oil capsules.

BREW YOUR AFTERNOON GREEN TEA

For greater hydration, brew a lot of green tea (decaf is always fine) in a little water—eight bags at a time in 1 cup of hot water. Let it sit for a few minutes, add ice, then drink it within the hour.

REDUCE YOUR SITTING TIME

To help lower your setpoint, spend less time sitting and more time moving around. After being seated at your computer or at your desk, get up and go for a walk around the office. If you want to try something a bit more energizing, consider a stand-up desk. Also, stand through meetings or phone calls whenever possible.

2:00 p.m.–4:00 p.m.
HAVE A MIDAFTERNOON SNACK (MEAL #4—OPTIONAL)

Have 1 SANE Meal Smoothie (NSVs and NDP) or 1 CLEAN high-prebiotic fiber and protein bar plus 1 SANE All-Veggie Smoothie. Also, take 1 teaspoon of pharmaceutical-grade cod liver oil.

DAILY SELF-COMPASSION MEDITATION FOR WEEK 1: THE COMPASSIONATE BODY SCAN

You may do your meditations at any time during the day that suits your schedule. If you struggle with a case of the blahs in the afternoon or are prone to afternoon snacking, doing your meditation after lunch can help you recenter and refocus.

Week 1's meditation is a compassionate body scan. Set up in your meditation position of choice and get settled.

2. The Practice

In this practice you will be bringing your attention and focus to your body, part by part. Start with your toes, then move into the soles of the feet, the heels of the feet, the shins, the calves, the knees, the thighs, the pelvis, the belly, the rib cage, the fingertips, the forearms, the elbows, the armpits, the collarbones, the neck and throat, the jaw, the muscles in your cheeks, the eyeballs, the forehead, the scalp, the ears, the skull. Try to go as slowly as you can, noticing as many sensations as possible. For example, does a certain body part feel heavy or light? Is there any pain or discomfort? What emotions seem to rise up for that body part? Can you feel the touch of the floor, or your clothing, or the air? If you notice tension, discomfort, or negative emotions, place a hand on your heart, breathe deeply, and return to focusing on the simple sensations of your physical body.

4:00 p.m.–6:00 p.m.

DO SANE ACTIVITY

Depending on what time you finish work, now is a good time to build activity into your routine. (You may also do SANE activity in the morning or during your lunch hour, depending on your personal schedule and preferences.)

This activity could be:

- Taking a restorative class such as yoga, Pilates, tai chi, or stretching.
- Going for a bike ride for 20 to 30 minutes.
- Taking a walk, preferably outside in nature, ideally with a person or animal that you like, for 20 to 30 minutes.

During the first week of the plan, you will want to start practicing eccentric exercise movements, as well as SANE interval training.

Review Chapters 12 and 13 for instructions on performing SANE activities.

6:00 p.m.–8:00 p.m.

EAT A SANE DINNER (MEAL #5)

Enjoy a recipe such as Dijon Salmon for dinner. This counts as your serving of ONDP. (The recipe is in Appendix A.) It makes 4 servings, so you may have some left over, or you could double the recipe and enjoy leftovers for lunch or dinner the next day. Along with it, have 1 to 2 servings of SANE Optimal Veggie Soup or smoothie. If you do not eat salmon or other optimal seafood, take 1 teaspoon of pharmaceutical-grade cod liver oil or a double dose of fish oil capsules.

Drink at least 16 ounces of water or green tea with the meal, assuming you are eating at least 2 hours before going to bed. The closer it gets to bedtime, the less you will want to drink to prevent bathroom breaks from interrupting your essential 8 hours of sleep.

Reminder: If this was one of your smarter exercise days, substitute the following for your fifth meal:

- 8-ounce sweet potato (you can season with anything natural and noncaloric such as salt or cinnamon, but no butter or oil)
- 1 to 2 servings SANE Optimal Veggie Soup or smoothie
- If you are still hungry, have 4 ounces of additional sweet potato.

TAKE YOUR NUTRACEUTICALS WITH DINNER

If you are using nutraceuticals, take some of them now. (You will be taking them in divided dosages each day—at breakfast, lunch, and dinner—to maximize their absorption.)

BATCH COOK (AT LEAST ON THE WEEKENDS)

On your weekends, purchase all your necessary SANE foods and ingredients at the grocery store and do any meal prep (like chopping vegetables) ahead of time. Make big batches of SANE dishes on the weekend and freeze a lot of it. At least, every time you cook, prepare two meals: one you will eat now and one you will eat later. Maybe even take this step further: create four meals every time you cook: one that you enjoy immediately, another that you enjoy the next day, and two meals' worth that you can freeze and enjoy the following week. Then, even if you feel tired after work, you'll be prepared to whip up a great SANE meal.

8:00 p.m.–10:30 p.m.
MAKE TIME FOR REFLECTION

Benjamin Franklin's day always ended with asking and answering this question: "What good have I done today?"

Asking and answering this important question at the end of your day gives you a chance to reflect and celebrate your day's achievements. It also helps you consider whether you are on target for reaching your goals.

At the end of each day, write in your journal or a notebook all of the positive things that happened during the course of that day. For example:

> The best part of my day so far was making SANE food choices, helping my team at work solve a problem, contributing to my SANE support group, receiving a compliment and encouragement from my boss, doing an errand for my neighbor, making a donation to a cause I believe in, or volunteering for a needed project, and so forth.

TAKE ZMA PRIOR TO BEDTIME

If you have opted to take ZMA, the usual recommended daily dosage is to take 3 capsules daily for men and 2 capsules daily for women, preferably on an empty stomach 30 to 60 minutes before bedtime.

FOCUS ON QUALITY SLEEP

I know this seems like common sense, but sleep is critical to lowering your setpoint. Maybe in the past you have been told to wake up at 4:00 a.m. and jog for an hour to lose weight. Well, that is like telling someone who just broke an ankle to stop icing it and to go jump up and down.

A broken metabolism really is like a broken ankle: *It heals itself* when you put less stress on it—not more. Sleeping less increases stress. Traditional exercise increases stress. Starvation increases stress. That's why every night, enjoy quality sleep.

You can sleep your way to a lower setpoint by removing many of the obstacles that prevent a lot of people from getting a good night's rest. Some suggestions:

- Stop using technology such as your cell phone, laptop, or computer at least 1 hour prior to bedtime.
- Create a calm sleep environment by darkening your room (absence of light helps raise sleep-inducing melatonin levels).
- Turn your LED alarm clock to the wall (because of the light).

- Limit any caffeine consumption to early in the day, if at all.
- Meditate, take a warm bath, or read a good book to help you relax and get ready for bed.
- Keep your bedroom cool (around 65 to 68 degrees).
- Get a foam roller and massage your muscles for 5 minutes before bed.
- Set a consistent bedtime, rather than varying your routine every night. Consistency helps prepare your body and your mind for a restful night's sleep. So for best results, try to maintain the same sleep schedule every day (even on weekends).
- Take ZMA.

Medication Management and Your Setpoint

If you feel like you are struggling with an extremely stubborn elevated setpoint, it could be a side effect of medication you're taking. This is common with antidepressants, mood stabilizers, insulin therapy, and birth control pills. All of these can raise your setpoint, interfere with your metabolism, and trigger weight gain.

If your antidepressant, antipsychotic, or antianxiety medication (SSRIs in particular) is adding pounds, work with your psychiatrist to find an alternative treatment plan that will keep weight gain to a minimum. Also, SANE living has a profound positive impact on brain chemistry, so you will want to work with your psychiatrist no matter what while transitioning to a SANE lifestyle.

If you have type 2 diabetes and are on insulin therapy, work directly with your primary care physician to monitor your blood sugar. With insulin therapy, it is believed that, as blood sugar comes under control with insulin, the metabolism adapts by slowing down. A vicious circle can be initiated as the extra weight gained stimulates insulin resistance, which in turn requires greater doses of insulin. Similar to its positive impact on mood, SANE living will radically improve blood sugar control, so it is essential to work with your physician here no matter what.

Prolonged use of birth control pills can usually cause weight gain due to their hormonal impact. Ask your primary care physician to evaluate the impact your form of birth control may have on your hormones and thus your setpoint, and suggest alternative strategies.

TIP

Be sure to get your free checklists, trackers, worksheets, and journals at SANESolution.com. They will make every day of the program much simpler, and I promise—and studies support (Hollis et al. 2008)—that by using these free tools daily, you will enjoy better and faster results.

WEEK 2—SAMPLE DAY

6:00 a.m.–8:00 a.m.

WAKE UP

Be consistent with your wake-up times: try to get up at the same time each morning, even on weekends. These make mornings easier to handle and get your day off to a positive start.

EAT A SANE BREAKFAST (MEAL #1)

Arrange a plate of smoked salmon and serve it with capers and some slices of red onion (this meal is your ONDP).

Fix a SANE All-Veggie Green Smoothie to enjoy with your breakfast (or, ideally, simply pick up one you batch prepared over the weekend). If you didn't previously batch blend, make three now, enjoy them on the go throughout your day, and add to your non-starchy vegetable goals. For information on how to make SANE smoothies, see Chapter 7.

Drink at least 16 ounces of water or green tea with the meal.

TAKE YOUR NUTRACEUTICALS WITH BREAKFAST

If you are using nutraceuticals, take some of them now. (You will be taking them in divided dosages each day—at breakfast, lunch, and dinner—to maximize their absorption.) If your ONDP is not seafood, take 1 teaspoon of pharmaceutical-grade cod liver oil or a double dose of fish oil capsules.

BREW YOUR MORNING GREEN TEA

For greater hydration, brew a lot of green tea in a little water—eight bags at a time in 12 ounces of hot water. Let it sit for a few minutes, add ice, then drink it within the hour. Do this once in the morning and once in the afternoon, and you are good to go.

BATCH PREP SMOOTHIES

Make two smoothies to take to work with you. Go to the recipe section, select a smoothie, and double the recipes. Divide your smoothies into plastic containers and refrigerate them as soon as you get to work. Reblend, or shake up, each smoothie prior to drinking it.

PRACTICE GRATITUDE

Once again, select two or three things, big or small, for which you are grateful. You will be surprised to find that this activity cancels out most of your anxiety and negativity about starting your day. Or go over your gratitude list. Add to it, if you can.

CREATE YOUR PLAN TO OVERCOME OBSTACLES
AND ACHIEVE YOUR GOAL

Think about how successfully you've been achieving your daily process goals. Are your emotions and mind-set shifting toward the positive? Positive thoughts and emotions drive you forward; they give you momentum. So if there's a bump in the road, you cruise right over it.

To continue that positive momentum, write out your process goals, broken down into Action Steps and Consistency Steps, along with your implementation intentions. Some additional examples for today, or this week:

I want to drink a gallon of SANE fluids, including water (Action Step) each day this week (Consistency Step). If I have a craving for coffee in the midafternoon, then I will drink a glass or two of water.

Or:

I will purchase a set of resistance bands (Action Step) on Monday after work so that I can practice eccentric training on Tuesday and Saturday this week (Consistency Step). If I work late on Tuesday, then I will identify available time slots on Wednesday that I can use to practice my eccentric training.

Or:

I will replace one of my normal snacks with a SANE All-Veggie Smoothie (Action Step) each day this week (Consistency Step). If I feel busy and hurried during my workweek, then I will prepare batches of SANE smoothies on Monday and Wednesday that I can take to work and shake or reblend when I am ready to drink them.

Or:

I will eat SANE meals (Action Step) each day this weekend, from Friday through Sunday (Consistency Step). If I am invited to a party, then I will eat a SANE dinner prior to going.

Also, formulate a possible replacement for any habits and routines you want to change. An example for today, or this week:

I will replace my negative habit of late-night eating with a positive habit. The cue is the time (9:00 p.m.) and the fact that I feel hungry (physical sensation). The routine is automatically going to the kitchen and choosing something to eat. The reward is the comfort and temporary lift I get from eating. I can replace the habit and the routine by fixing a SANE snack such as a handful of raw nuts at 9:00 p.m. when I feel hungry (new routine), and this will satisfy my hunger.

Other strategies for replacing this habit include: making sure I eat at least three SANE meals during the day, removing inSANE foods from my house, and replacing the late-night snack habit with something that keeps me busy in the hours prior to bedtime, such as reading or working on a home project (this will be helpful if my snacking is more of a mindless habit than actual hunger).

Also for this week: If you feel like you are addicted to certain foods, select a food from which you want to free yourself this week. Decide which SANE substitution will help you do that. For example:

> The food I want to free myself from this week is cookies. The SANE
> substitution I can replace it with is to make SANE Almond Cookies
> and have them on hand when I want a cookie.

9:00 a.m.–11:00 a.m.

HYDRATE

Despite your morning SANE smoothie and green tea, you may be slightly dehydrated. To stay hydrated, consider drinking 1 or 2 glasses of water.

PLUG INTO YOUR ONLINE SUPPORT GROUP

Take 5 minutes this morning to access the SANE help center for support and information on new tips, tools, and tricks to help maximize your results.

HAVE A MIDMORNING SNACK (MEAL #2—OPTIONAL)

Have 1 SANE Meal Smoothie (NSVs and NDP) or 1 CLEAN high-prebiotic fiber and protein bar plus 1 SANE All-Veggie Smoothie. Also, take 1 teaspoon of pharmaceutical-grade cod liver oil.

12:00 p.m.–2:00 p.m.

EAT A SANE LUNCH (MEAL #3)

Arrange a serving of leftover Dijon Salmon or tuna (this is your ONDP) atop a generous bed of romaine lettuce. This lunch is also an example of one you can easily pack in the morning in a container to take to work. With your ONDP, have 1 to 2 servings of SANE Optimal Veggie Soup or smoothie.

Drink at least 16 ounces of water or green tea with the meal.

TAKE YOUR NUTRACEUTICALS WITH LUNCH

If you are using nutraceuticals, take some of them now. (You will be taking them in divided dosages each day—at breakfast, lunch, and dinner—to maximize their absorption.) If your ONDP is not seafood, take 1 teaspoon of pharmaceutical-grade cod liver oil or a double dose of fish oil capsules.

BREW YOUR AFTERNOON GREEN TEA

For greater hydration, brew a lot of green tea in a little water—eight bags at a time in 1 cup of hot water. Let it sit for a few minutes, add ice, then drink within the hour.

REDUCE YOUR SITTING TIME

Be sure to get up from your office chair and move around frequently, or talk on your phone while standing up. Some additional suggestions this week:

- Use a two-way speakerphone or quality headset so you can be more mobile while you are on the phone.
- Rather than call or email coworkers, walk over to their desks. Stand in your colleagues' office to discuss things, or take a walk to chat.
- Make frequent trips to the watercooler or water fountain. As a bonus, this is a way to increase the amount of water you drink.

2:00 p.m.–4:00 p.m.
HAVE A MIDAFTERNOON SNACK (MEAL #4—OPTIONAL)

Have 1 SANE Meal Smoothie (NSVs and NDP) or 1 CLEAN high-prebiotic fiber and protein bar plus 1 SANE All-Veggie Smoothie. Also, take 1 teaspoon of pharmaceutical-grade cod liver oil.

DAILY SELF-COMPASSION MEDITATION FOR WEEK 2: AFFECTIONATE BREATHING

The practice: Take a few moments to do a quick body scan and notice any sensations. After all the compassionate body scanning practice you did last week, this should be pretty familiar. Take three deep breaths to release any tension. Then allow your breathing to return to normal softly and evenly in through the nose and out through the nose. Notice the sensation of the breath in and out of your body. Is it raggedy? Is it smooth? Where do you notice the breath the most in your body? In your throat? On the backside of your rib cage? Deep in your belly? In your pelvis? Just keep bringing the focus back to the inhale and the exhale. After several minutes of noticing the breath, in and out, let your lips soften into a half smile. With every breath you take in, imagine you are breathing in affection and kindness toward yourself. And with every exhale, breathe out affection and kindness to others. Keep bringing your mind back to the intention of affection and kindness, in and out. No judgment if your mind wanders! Just bring it back to affection and kindness, in toward yourself, out toward others.

4:00 p.m.–6:00 p.m.

DO SANE ACTIVITY

Depending on when you finish work, now is a good time to build activity into your routine. (Remember, too, that you may also do SANE activity in the morning or during your lunch hour, depending on your personal schedule and preferences.)

This activity could be:

- Taking a restorative class such as yoga, Pilates, tai chi, or stretching.
- Going for a bike ride for 20 to 30 minutes.
- Taking a walk, preferably outside in nature, for 20 to 30 minutes.
- Practicing eccentric exercise movements for 10 minutes, once a week.
- Performing 10 minutes of SANE interval training, once a week.

Review Chapters 12 and 13 for instructions on performing SANE activities.

6:00 p.m.–8:00 p.m.

EAT A SANE DINNER (MEAL #5)

Enjoy Bayou Shrimp for dinner (the recipe is in Appendix A). This counts as a serving of NDP. Alternatively, you can have white meat chicken or lean beef. With your nutrient-dense protein, have 1 to 2 servings of SANE Optimal Veggie Soup or smoothie.

Drink at least 16 ounces of water or green tea with the meal.

TAKE YOUR NUTRACEUTICALS WITH DINNER

If you are using nutraceuticals, take some of them now. (You will be taking them in divided dosages each day—at breakfast, lunch, and dinner—to maximize their absorption.) If your ONDP is not seafood, take 1 teaspoon of pharmaceutical-grade cod liver oil or a double dose of fish oil capsules.

Reminder: If today was one of your smarter exercise days, substitute the following for your fifth meal:

- 8-ounce sweet potato (you can season with anything natural and noncaloric such as salt or cinnamon, but no butter or oil)
- 1 to 2 servings SANE Optimal Veggie Soup or smoothie
- If you are still hungry, have 4 ounces of additional sweet potato.

8:00 p.m.—10:30 p.m.

MAKE TIME FOR REFLECTION

Ask and answer the question "What was the best part of my day?" or "What good have I done today?" Write, in your journal or a notebook, the best part or parts of your day.

TAKE ZMA PRIOR TO BEDTIME

If you have opted to take ZMA, the usual recommended daily dosage is to take 3 capsules daily for men and 2 capsules daily for women, preferably on an empty stomach 30 to 60 minutes before bedtime.

FOCUS ON QUALITY SLEEP

Be sure that this week, you have removed as many obstacles to quality sleep as you can. Also, try to go to bed at roughly the same time every night, even on weekends.

WEEK 3—SAMPLE DAY

6:00 a.m.–8:00 a.m.

WAKE UP

By week 3, you are probably quite consistent with your wake-up times. Keeping regular bedtimes and wake-up times will leave you more refreshed.

EAT A SANE BREAKFAST (MEAL #1)

With your ONDP, have 1 to 2 servings of SANE Optimal Veggie Soup or smoothie. Also, drink at least 16 ounces of water or green tea with the meal.

TAKE YOUR NUTRACEUTICALS WITH BREAKFAST

If you are using nutraceuticals, take some of them now. (You will be taking them in divided dosages each day—at breakfast, lunch, and dinner—to maximize their absorption.) If your ONDP is not seafood, take 1 teaspoon of pharmaceutical-grade cod liver oil or a double dose of fish oil capsules.

BREW YOUR MORNING GREEN TEA

For greater hydration, brew a lot of green tea in a little water—eight bags at a time in 1 cup of hot water. Let it sit for a few minutes, add ice, then drink within the hour. Do this once in the morning and once in the afternoon, and you are good to go.

PRACTICE GRATITUDE

Once again, select two or three things, big or small, for which you are grateful. You will be surprised to find that this activity cancels out most of your anxiety and negativity about starting your day. Or go over your gratitude list. Add to it, if you can.

CREATE YOUR PLAN TO OVERCOME OBSTACLES AND ACHIEVE YOUR GOAL

This week, continue to write out your process goals, broken down into Action Steps and Consistency Steps, along with your implementation intentions. Some additional examples for today or this week:

> I will buy groceries in bulk over the weekend (Action Step) and pack SANE lunches for work on Monday, Tuesday, Wednesday, Thursday, and Friday this week (Consistency Step) in place of going out to eat or getting fast food. If I do not have time to pack lunch on any

given day, then I will walk over to the salad restaurant around the corner and fix myself a SANE salad with lots of green vegetables, raw salad vegetables, and a nutrient-dense protein such as eggs or ham from the salad bar.

Or:

I will sign up for yoga classes (Action Step) and attend two classes this week (Consistency Step) to reduce my stress level and increase my time spent in restorative activities. If I have to unexpectedly go out of town on business this week, then I will pack resistance bands in my suitcase and do eccentric exercises...or make reservations in a hotel with a swimming pool or gym...or walk the halls/climb stairs in my hotel.

Or:

I will handle stress better this week so I will extend my self-compassion meditation time to 20 minutes (Action Step) and practice it three times this week (Consistency Step). If I feel anxious or want to eat emotionally, then I will do deep breathing, and/or I will contact my support group or my SANE Certified Coach.

Continue to work on habit replacement this week. Formulate a possible replacement for any habits and routines you want to change. An example for today, or this week:

I will replace my habit of going to Starbucks every morning to get a latte and Danish with a positive habit. My cue is the time of day—morning. Getting a latte and Danish is my routine. My reward could be any number of things: the rush from the latte and Danish, or maybe it is the chance to socialize. So when I go to Starbucks, I will change my routine there. Instead of the latte and Danish, I will get just coffee or green tea, then I will socialize for 10 minutes. Or I will change my routine entirely by going for a walk in the morning.

Also for this week: If you still feel like you are addicted to certain foods, select a food from which you want to free yourself. Decide which SANE substitution will help you do that. For example:

The food I want to free myself from this week is pasta. The SANE substitution I will replace it with is spaghetti squash or zoodles (spiralized zucchini) and top it with sugar-free pasta sauce, mixed with cooked lean ground beef.

SLOW-COOK TONIGHT'S SANE MEAL

Here is something you can do just about any day of the week during this 21-Day Plan: Put SANE nutrient-dense proteins, non-starchy veggies, and spices of your choice in a slow cooker with a little liquid. Adjust the setting to low, and dinner will be ready when you arrive home. Try Slow Cooker Tomato & Herb Beef, for example (the recipe is in Appendix A).

9:00 a.m.–11:00 a.m.

HYDRATE

Despite your morning SANE smoothie and green tea, you may be slightly dehydrated. To stay hydrated, consider downing one or two glasses of water.

PLUG INTO YOUR ONLINE SUPPORT GROUP

Take 5 minutes this morning to access the SANE help center for support and information on new tips, tools, and tricks to help maximize your results.

HAVE A MIDMORNING SNACK (MEAL #2—OPTIONAL)

Have 1 SANE Meal Smoothie (NSVs and NDP) or 1 CLEAN high-prebiotic fiber and protein bar plus 1 SANE All-Veggie Smoothie. Also, take 1 teaspoon of pharmaceutical-grade cod liver oil.

12:00 p.m.–2:00 p.m.

EAT A SANE LUNCH (MEAL #3)

Take any dinner leftovers to work and heat them up for lunch! With your ONDP, have 1 to 2 servings of SANE Optimal Veggie Soup or smoothie.

Drink at least 16 ounces of water or green tea with the meal.

TAKE YOUR NUTRACEUTICALS WITH LUNCH

If you are using nutraceuticals, take some of them now. (You will be taking them in divided dosages each day—at breakfast, lunch, and dinner—to maximize their absorption.) If your ONDP is not seafood, take 1 teaspoon of pharmaceutical-grade cod liver oil or a double dose of fish oil capsules.

BREW YOUR AFTERNOON GREEN TEA

For greater hydration, brew a lot of green tea in a little water—eight bags at a time in 1 cup of hot water. Let it sit for a few minutes, add ice, then drink within the hour.

REDUCE YOUR SITTING TIME

Be sure to get up from your office chair and move around frequently, or talk on your phone while standing up. Some additional suggestions:

- Do a lap around your floor. Go outside. Get some tea.
- During presentations and meetings, stand as much as possible.
- Take the stairs. Instead of riding the elevator or escalator, step it up a notch and take the stairs.
- Set a timer on your phone that signals you to stand up and stretch and move around every hour.

2:00 p.m.–4:00 p.m.
HAVE A MIDAFTERNOON SNACK (MEAL #4—OPTIONAL)

Have 1 SANE Meal Smoothie (NSVs and NDP) or 1 CLEAN high-prebiotic fiber and protein bar plus 1 SANE All-Veggie Smoothie. Also, take 1 teaspoon of pharmaceutical-grade cod liver oil.

DAILY SELF-COMPASSION MEDITATION FOR WEEK 3: LOVING-KINDNESS

The practice: Begin by bringing awareness into the present moment. Note any sensations in the body, any sounds around you, and your breath. Next take your attention to something about yourself that brings you emotional pain. Allow that feeling and any other feelings associated with it to surface. Where do you experience these emotions in your body? Allow these feelings to just be wherever they happen to be in the body. Place both hands over your heart, and silently say: *May I be safe. May I be kind to myself. May I be healthy and strong. May I accept myself as I am.* Start with these phrases and repeat. As you get more and more practice at this, you can choose your own loving-kindness phrases to repeat.

4:00 p.m.–6:00 p.m.

DO SANE ACTIVITY

In your third week, perform your full 10-minute eccentric routine 1 day a week, and your full 10-minute SANE interval training on another day. You're investing only 20 minutes a week in your body's development—which frees you up for the real world and eliminates the stress of deadlines, errands, and other commitments. Here is a look at how to schedule both into your week:

Monday: 10 minutes of SANE eccentric training
Tuesday: Relax and recover
Wednesday: Relax and recover
Thursday: 10 minutes of SANE interval training
Friday: Relax and recover
Saturday: Relax and recover
Sunday: Relax and recover

Please push yourself as hard as you safely can and then continue to push yourself more and more gradually by adding resistance at least every other workout. As you improve the quality of your health and fitness, you must improve the quality of your activity to keep progressing. Think about training your body as you would think about training your mind. Once you've mastered multiplication tables, for example, move on to something more challenging to maximize your mental capacity. The same thing goes for your body. Keep adding resistance and challenging yourself to maximize your physical capacity. See Chapter 12 for more information on working out at home.

You may also continue to do restorative activity this week, such as yoga, Pilates, tai chi, stretching, walking in nature, or bike riding.

HAVE A SANE SMOOTHIE AFTER YOUR WORKOUT

After either your SANE eccentric workout or SANE interval training, prepare a SANE smoothie that includes a scoop or two of clean whey protein. After a workout, your muscles require an immediate supply of amino acids to start the repair and rebuilding process. Clean whey protein is rich in leucine, which is essential for muscle development because it turns on the process of muscle protein synthesis and supplies critical building blocks for muscle protein. Whey is the perfect protein to consume after a workout because its amino acids are discharged rapidly.

6:00 p.m.–8:00 p.m.

EAT A SANE DINNER (MEAL #5)

Since you exercised smarter today, you'll leverage the SANE sweet potato substitution. Bake, microwave, or reheat 8 ounces of sweet potato and enjoy it seasoned with anything natural and noncaloric such as salt or cinnamon. Avoid adding butter and oil. Also enjoy 1 to 2 servings of a SANE Optimal Veggie Soup or smoothie. Wait 10 minutes after eating those and if you are still hungry, have 4 ounces of additional sweet potato.

If done no more than twice per week and on days when you exercise smarter, during these 21 days only, the specific form of starch found in sweet potatoes eaten at this specific quantity at this specific time helps to optimize your metabolic rate, thyroid hormone output, sympathetic nervous system activity, appetite hormones, and sex hormones.

TAKE YOUR NUTRACEUTICALS WITH DINNER

If you are using nutraceuticals, take some of them now. (You will be taking them in divided dosages each day—at breakfast, lunch, and dinner—to maximize their absorption.) If your ONDP is not seafood, take 1 teaspoon of pharmaceutical-grade cod liver oil or a double dose of fish oil capsules.

8:00 p.m.–10:30 p.m.

MAKE TIME FOR REFLECTION

Ask and answer the question "What was the best part of my day?" or "What good have I done today?" In your journal or a notebook, write the best part or parts of your day.

Now that you've gone through week 3 of the plan, you've made amazing progress. Reflect upon it here. For example, write about how you feel better about yourself—and how this has improved your life. Also, write about how eating more and exercising less has had a positive impact on your life. Spend no more than 15 minutes completing this work—at least once a week. Think of it as a written meditation. Let your thoughts flow freely and enjoy the exercise. For example:

> Since living SANEly for 3 weeks, I feel younger and more energetic. I can accomplish more during the day than ever before, because I am not dragging, physically or mentally. Best of all, I have lost 10 pounds! I am starting to fit in clothes I haven't worn for years, and I feel sexy and attractive. My relationship with my spouse is better—more loving and more understanding—because I love myself more and feel good about where I am in life. I'm excited about going forward.

TAKE ZMA PRIOR TO BEDTIME

If you have opted to take ZMA, the usual recommended daily dosage is to take 3 capsules daily for men and 2 capsules daily for women, preferably on an empty stomach 30 to 60 minutes before bedtime.

FOCUS ON QUALITY SLEEP

Be sure that this week, you have removed as many obstacles to quality sleep as you can. Also, try to go to bed at roughly the same time every night, even on weekends.

What can I say right now except—congratulations! You have turned 21 days into a keystone physical and mental transformation for yourself because of your brave decision to make a better life for yourself. Opening the door to SANE living and making a commitment to do something you've never done before has made you leaner, stronger, and more passionate about life. You've done it without feeling the least bit deprived or overexercised. You have worked hard at changing your body and mind to unlock that naturally thin person inside you. In so many ways, you have honored yourself beyond measure.

I know this is the end of the 21 days, but it's really just the beginning. You will only get better at SANE living. In the next and final chapter, I will show you how to enjoy a lower setpoint for the rest of your life by being #SANE4Life.

SANE Points

- Supercharge your motivation by seeing these 21 days the same way you'd see the first 21 days after a major surgery, making this your number-one priority and committing to it 100 percent.
- Following a SANE routine each day keeps you functioning at the highest level possible in all three areas of your life—mind, body, and spirit. It makes you a better, more positive person. It gets you to a lower setpoint and a healthier weight.
- Once you start eating and exercising SANEly, they'll start to feel natural, if not necessary, for your new lifestyle.
- Keep incorporating SANE mind-set activities—goal-setting, habit change, loving support, meditation, and gratitude journaling—into your daily life, and you will experience a remarkable transformation.
- These 21 days are not the end; they are the beginning!

CHAPTER 16

#SANE4Life

Regardless of what the scale or magazines say, I hope you see a beautiful person in the mirror right now.

Regardless of what happened in your past, I hope you see tremendous possibility and hope in your future.

Regardless of how many times you have yo-yo'ed, I hope you are courageously choosing to lower your setpoint.

Regardless of how many quick fixes disappointed you previously, I hope you are giving yourself the gift of patient persistence presently.

Regardless of how discouraged you felt after your last doctor visit, I hope you see that you can control your cholesterol, diabetes, blood sugar, and insulin.

Regardless of how ashamed you've been made to feel in the past, I hope you now realize how truly miraculous you are.

Regardless of how many mind-numbing food lists and complex conditions you previously believed are required to lose weight, I hope you are unlocking the proven setpoint-lowering power of simple SANEity and unconditional self-love.

Regardless of how insane modern life becomes, I hope you continue to take this road less traveled, because as Robert Frost told us: "It will make all the difference."

If you are reading this chapter after doing the 21-Day Plan exactly as prescribed, then you are well on your way to successfully lowering your setpoint; healing your brain, gut, hormones, and metabolism; reclaiming your health; adopting a new empowering mind-set; and officially regaining your sanity and SANEity. Congratulations! You have put in the work, and it shows.

Because you have made it this far down this infinitely more enjoyable, empowering, and slimming road, it's time to let you in on something I don't share with many people. You see, over the course of the past 3 weeks, you have been doing more than just transforming your mind and your body and lowering your setpoint as a result. You have been entering a state of being that we here at SANE call "nutritional serenity." What exactly does that mean? It means freedom from calorie counting, rigid meal plans, yo-yo dieting, scales, laps and miles, food obsessions and cravings—the list really could go on and on and on.

Think back to life prior to going SANE. What was your life truly like? You and I both know you'd never choose to go back. In fact, our most successful members consistently tell us that they *can't* go back. Why? Because learning how to lower your setpoint and learning how to see yourself, food, fitness, and life through a SANE lens is like learning to read. It's like becoming literate after decades of struggling with illiteracy. Once you learn it, the world never looks the same again. And of course, you'd never go back, because you have so much more power and possibility now.

It helps to think of SANE as "wellness literacy." Once you "get it," so much confusion is *instantly* replaced with clarity. You will never return to the starvation, shame, and stress. You will never be hungry or feel deprived again. You will never need to spend hours exercising. All of that is gone and has been replaced with peace with your body, peace with food, and peace with yourself.

With this peace, you now can take care of the things in your life that actually matter—because you will no longer be saddled by constant shame, guilt, or worry over your weight. No one is going to say at your funeral, "Kelly had really defined abs." They are going to say, "Kelly was a truly beautiful person who blessed everyone she met. She made the world a better place and enhanced the lives of everyone she interacted with." Meaning and purpose in life—that is really the essence of nutritional serenity. And empowering you to live that life is why we are here.

So the question is: Where do you go from here? Well, we call it #SANE4Life. Because you now have a loving, committed, and stable relationship with food. It's just how you naturally and effortlessly live your life now. SANEity is your new normal, and any bumps in the road are smoothed out automatically by your lower setpoint. You have the tools, the awareness, and the information to go forward in confidence and self-love that you can do this for the rest of your life. Let's look at how this all works.

#SANE4LIFE

The cornerstone for lowering your setpoint and rediscovering the naturally thin person inside you has been SANE nutrition, and the cornerstone to sustaining your lower setpoint long-term is also SANE nutrition. After your first 21-day cycle, you can choose to either continue with another cycle of the setpoint-lowering plan (which will reduce your setpoint by another 10 pounds in 21 days) or shift to #SANE4Life.

This is as simple as staying so full of non-starchy vegetables, nutrient-dense protein, whole-food fats, and low-fructose fruits—in that order—that you rarely have room for inSANE processed starches, sweets, and trans fats. When eating out, pass on the pasta and rice and ask your server to hold the starch but double the vegetables. At home, skip the rolls and enjoy a larger helping of a protein-packed main course and two or three extra helpings of non-starchy vegetables.

When selecting which foods to make you feel most alive, choose those that are "most alive." For example, pasta that has been sitting on a shelf for a year is far from alive. A bag of organic cane sugar is a bag of death in more ways than one. Compare that to a bag of leafy green non-starchy vegetables that are currently alive, or scrumptious salmon that was alive a couple of days ago. You will still take the paint-by-numbers approach to your plate, which will look like "Your Sane Plate" in Chapter 8.

As you already learned, within the primary SANE food groups of non-starchy vegetables, nutrient-dense protein, whole-food fats, and low-fructose fruits, there are optimal options that will fast-track your progress. All the food listed below provides common examples. They are not exhaustive. There are way too many SANE food options to list them all!

Non-starchy Vegetables (10+ Servings per Day)

OPTIMAL (deep green leafy veggies)	NORMAL (veggies you could eat raw)
Alfalfa, arugula, bok choy, barley grass, Brussels sprouts, chard, garlic, greens, kale, kelp, mixed greens, moringa, neem, romaine lettuce, seaweed, spinach, spirulina, watercress, wheat grass	Alfalfa sprouts, artichoke, asparagus, bean sprouts, beets, bell peppers, broccoli, cabbage, carrots, cauliflower, celery, cucumber, eggplant, endive, green beans, leeks, mushrooms, onion, peppers, squash, sugar snap peas, tomatoes, zucchini

If raw and leafy, a serving is the size of two of your fists. If raw and not leafy, a serving is the size of your fist. If cooked, a serving is a little smaller than the size of your fist.

Most people stop eating naturally at about 3 servings in a single sitting. It is practically impossible to overeat non-starchy vegetables. You would get too full.

Examples of a single serving of non-starchy vegetables:

- 3 cups of raw leafy green vegetables
- 6 asparagus spears
- 8 baby carrots
- 5 broccoli florets
- 1 Roma tomato
- 4 slices of onion
- 5 cherry tomatoes
- 5 sticks of celery
- 1 whole carrot
- ½ cup of cooked spinach
- 1 tablespoon whole-food veggie powder

Nutrient-Dense Protein (3 to 6 Servings per Day)

Important Note for Vegetarians and Anyone with Special Needs

#SANE4Life can be enjoyed along with any lifestyle such as vegetarian, paleo, and low-carb, and during any life stage. While your SANE Certified Coaches can provide one-on-one guidance on personalizing your SANEity, the short version is that everything here is a suggestion (not a requirement), and you can customize your menu to include the SANEst versions of foods compatible with your lifestyle. For example, a SANE vegetarian would NOT start eating meat. Rather, she would learn how to choose the SANEst vegetarian protein options.

OPTIMAL (shellfish, fatty fish, organ meats)	NORMAL (humanely raised seafood and proteins)
Oysters, clams, mussels, liver, salmon, sardines, anchovies, sea bass, tuna	Catfish; chicken; cod; cottage cheese; egg whites combined with whole eggs; flounder; grass-fed beef; ham; lamb; lean conventional beef; plain Greek yogurt; pork; 100 percent pure unflavored whey, pea, or rice protein concentrate with no additives; shrimp; snapper; squid (calamari); tilapia; trout; turkey

As a general rule of thumb, a food is a nutrient-dense protein if it's found directly in nature and more of its calories come from protein than from fat or carbohydrate (more info below). Exceptions include some low-sugar and low-fat dairy products and natural SANE protein powders/bars.

For best results, be sure to enjoy a total of about 30 grams of protein (about the size of a man's hand) *every* time you eat.

Determining if a food gets more of its calories from protein than from fat or carbohydrate is as easy as 1, 2, 3:

1. Look at the nutrition label and multiply the grams of protein in a serving by 4.
2. Divide that number by the number of calories in a serving.
3. Multiply by 100 and that's the percent of calories in the food from protein.

For example, consider a can of tuna. It contains 42 grams of protein and 191 total calories; 42 grams of protein times 4 calories per gram of protein equals 168 calories from protein; 168 divided by 191 total calories equals .88. Multiply that by 100 and you see that this tuna is 88 percent protein. Since calories come from protein, carbohydrate, and fat, if a food gets more than 50 percent of its calories from protein, it must be more protein than carbs or fat. Easy, protein-packed, and delicious!

Most people would stop eating naturally at 2 servings in a single sitting. Except men trying to "prove their manhood" at barbeques, it is practically impossible to overeat nutrient-dense protein. You would get uncomfortably full.

Examples of a single serving:

- 1 piece of humanely raised meat or fish about the size of your hand
- 1 heaping cup of cottage cheese or plain Greek yogurt

- 4 tablespoons of pure unflavored whey protein concentrate
- 1 whole egg + 5 egg whites
- 8 egg whites
- 1 can of tuna

Whole-Food Fats (3 to 6 Servings per Day)

OPTIMAL (uniquely nutritious)	NORMAL (eggs, raw nuts, and seeds)
Coconut, coconut milk, coconut flour, cocoa/cacao, cocoa/cacao nibs, avocado, flax seeds, chia seeds, macadamias, olives	Almonds, Brazil nuts, chestnuts, eggs, hazelnuts, hemp seeds, pecans, pistachios, pumpkin seeds, sunflower seeds, walnuts

As a general rule of thumb, a food is a whole-food fat if it's found directly in nature and more of its calories come from fat than from protein or carbohydrate. Determine this the same way you did for protein except multiply grams of fat per serving by 9 (since fat has 9 calories per gram...not 4, like protein).

For example, a large egg contains 5 grams of fat and 71 total calories; 5 grams of fat times 9 calories per gram of fat equals 45 calories from fat; 45 divided by 71 total calories equals .63. Multiply this by 100 and you see that an egg is 63 percent fat and is therefore a whole-food fat. Also note that two large eggs are a single serving of whole-food fats as together they contain a total of 142 calories.

A serving is about the size of your middle and pointer finger side by side. If the nuts are mashed into butter (i.e., natural nut butter), a serving is the size of your thumb. Two whole eggs are a serving. When combined with non-starchy vegetables and nutrient-dense protein, most people would stop eating naturally at 2 servings in a single sitting.

When in doubt, a serving of whole-food fats contains about 150 calories.

Examples of a single serving of less common whole-food fats:

- ½ cup coconut flour
- Unlimited cocoa
- 2 cups SANE coconut milk
- ¼ cup chia seeds
- ¼ cup chocolate bites/cacao nibs
- ¼ cup flax seeds

Low-Fructose Fruits (0 to 3 Servings per Day)

OPTIMAL (least sugar, most nutrition)	NORMAL (berries and citrus)
Acai berry, goji berry, noni fruit, purple aronia, mangosteen	Blackberries, blueberries, boysenberry, cranberries, cantaloupe, casaba melon, cherries, coconut water, grapefruit, guava, lemon, lime, nectarine, papaya, peaches, raspberries, rhubarb, strawberries

A serving is the size of your fist. Most people would stop eating naturally at 2 servings in a single sitting. It is practically impossible to overeat berries and citrus fruits. The food would become unappetizing. The first orange would be tasty. The second one would be good. The third one would be tiresome. The fourth wouldn't be appealing.

Examples of a single serving of low-fructose fruits:

- 6 strawberries
- 1 orange
- ½ grapefruit
- ½ cup blueberries

Legumes/Beans (0 to 1 Serving per Day)
A serving is the size of your fist.

Any Other Fruit (0 to 1 Serving per Day)
A serving is the size of your fist.

Any Other Dairy (0 to 1 Serving per Day)
A serving of butter is the size of the tip of your thumb (1 teaspoon). A serving of cheese is about the size of your thumb. A serving of milk and yogurt is 1 cup (8 ounces). Most people could easily eat 4 servings of butter or cheese but only a serving or two of milk or yogurt in a single sitting. Baked goods can be saturated with hidden butter. Every time anyone eats pizza, they are likely eating over 4 servings of cheese. Butter and cheese are easy to overeat.

Other Fats (0 to 1 Serving per Day)
A serving is a conventional fatty steak or dark meat that is the size of your hand. A tablespoon of oil is a serving. Coconut oil is the SANEst oil.

Barring men trying to "prove something," most people would stop eating fatty meat naturally at 2 servings in a single sitting. Yet it is extremely easy to over-eat oil. Eat anything fried and you will easily eat at least 4 servings of oil.

Starch/Starchy Vegetables (0 Servings per Day)

Serving sizes vary. The key point is that a serving of starch is small. For example, a medium bag of popcorn contains 8 servings. Starches are extremely easy to overeat because they are dry, relatively low in fiber, and protein poor. Most people overeat starch daily without knowing it. When ranchers want to fatten livestock, they stop feeding their cows non-starchy vegetables and start feeding them starch (generally corn).

> TIP: As a general rule, if it is not sweet, does not need to be refrigerated, and takes a long time to spoil, it likely fits in this group. If you can't find it directly in nature (i.e., there's no such thing as a bread bush) and it is not sweet, it likely fits in this group.

The number of starch servings in common foods:

- inSANE baked goods → 4 servings
- Baked potato → 3 servings
- French fries → 4 servings
- Pasta and rice → 4 servings

Sweets/Sweetened Drinks (0 Servings per Day)

Ten grams of sugar (i.e., anything with calories that is added to food to make it sweeter) is a serving. Sweets are the easiest food to overeat. Some sweeteners aren't even recognized as food by the body and never trigger a full feeling. This is why you can take in 3 servings of sweets by drinking a soda and still have plenty of room for a super-sized value meal. Traditional portions of sweets and sweetened drinks contain 3 to 8 servings of sweets. The fastest way to gain fat and damage your health is to eat and drink sweeteners.

NOTE: Natural noncaloric sweeteners such as stevia, erythritol, xylitol, and luo han guo do not count as a serving of anything. You can find these at most health food stores, Amazon, and SANESolution.com.

The number of sweetener servings in common foods:

- Can of soda → 3 servings
- Desserts → 4 servings
- Sweetened cereal → 4 servings
- Candy → 3 servings
- Store-bought fruit juice → 3 servings

It is perfectly reasonable to reach this point and say, "I do not always want to substitute non-starchy vegetables, nutrient-dense protein, and whole-food fats for starches and sweets the rest of my life." Don't worry—it's all good.

Amazing things have happened to you physically and psychologically that will help you stay the SANE course easily. The biggest benefit is that you have lowered your setpoint by healing your hormones, gut, brain, and metabolism—which allows you to *occasionally* enjoy some inSANE foods without undoing all the things you've achieved metabolically.

You see, your metabolic system is a lot like your immune system. If you have a healthy immune system and temporarily catch a cold, it's not the end of the world. Although you may feel sick for a short time, your immune system is still healthy. It will still work to resolve that problem over time. You can never avoid all bacteria and all viruses. That's not possible. What you can do is keep your immune system as healthy as possible so that when things do not go according to plan—with an invasion of viruses and bacteria, for example—you can recover quickly. Your metabolic system works the same way. If you have a healthy metabolic system, a little bit of inSANEity isn't going to break the system. The system is healed, so if you go a little bit inSANE, you will not gain 25 pounds overnight and your glucose and insulin levels aren't going to go out of whack overnight.

Plus, going SANE is all about progress, rather than perfection. Do your best to get the big things right, most of the time. You can burn as little or as much body fat as you want. You can stay in control by following these additional guidelines.

Try not to exceed 2 servings of starches and 1 serving of inSANE sweets daily. However, the fewer of these you eat, the slimmer you'll stay.

Eat inSANE dessert once a week (or not at all), and SANE desserts up to three times a week.

Enjoy one to three SANE smoothies a day.

Actively try to drink more water and green tea.

Use SANE substitutions as much as you can. Unless the food is 100 percent synthetic nonsense, SANESolution.com has a scrumptious setpoint-lowering substitution for it, including ice cream, cakes, and cookies. One of the coolest things about SANE eating is that every single flavor is available—sweet, salty, fatty, bitter—all of it; you just make SANE substitutions. You never need to be hungry or have cravings, because all flavors are available to you.

SANE ACTIVITY FOR LIFE MAINTENANCE

Staying active to maintain your improved health and lower setpoint is not much different than the physical activity you used to lower your setpoint. The important thing is to continue to move the way we have discussed in the three buckets of activity: eccentric resistance exercise, SANE intervals, and restorative activity. You still want to work out just as smart—to keep your setpoint low and metabolism in high gear and keep the weight off. SANE activity is essential to doing that.

To maintain your lower setpoint and ideal weight:

Continue your eccentric training. This type of activity, as you recall, triggers a very specific hormonal response that helps you maintain your lower setpoint. It is the super-specific exercise prescription to heal your metabolism as efficiently as possible that literally anyone can do and can be done for the rest of your life.

Remember to continue using more resistance than you can lift and focusing on the lowering portion of an exercise and performing it slowly.

All you still need is a 10-minute eccentric workout a week. Work on increasing your resistance, perhaps with weights or weight machines at a gym. At SANESolution.com, you can also find videos that show you how to perform eccentric training on dumbbells and kettlebells—and do so by increasing resistance.

Continue your SANE interval training on a stationary bike. In addition to your eccentric workouts, keep performing all-out intervals that require quick energy. Intervals are an excellent strategy for weight maintenance, since research shows this type of training burns energy for days after, despite the brief time (10 minutes) spent doing the actual intervals.

Pursue restorative activity. If you haven't tried restorative exercise, such as yoga, Pilates, tai chi, and other meditative-type activities, please give them a shot. They are excellent at reducing stress and curbing food cravings.

Yoga is a particularly good choice for weight maintenance. A 2005 study led by researchers at Fred Hutchinson Cancer Research Center in Seattle discovered that a regular yoga practice prevented middle-age normal-weight adults from gaining weight and promoted weight loss in those who are overweight. Published in *Alternative Therapies in Health and Medicine*, this study was the first of its kind to measure the effects of yoga on weight (Kristal 2005).

The researchers recruited 15,500 healthy men and women between the ages of 45 and 55 who were asked to complete a written questionnaire recalling their physical activity (including yoga) and weight history. The study measured the impact of yoga with weight change, independent of other factors such as diet or other types of physical activity.

The researchers found that between the ages of 45 and 55, most people gained about a pound a year. However, the adults who were of normal weight at age 45 and regularly practiced yoga gained about 3 fewer pounds during that 10-year period than those who didn't do yoga. For the study, regular yoga practice was defined as practicing at least 30 minutes once a week for 4 or more years. The men and women who were overweight and did yoga lost about 5 pounds, while those who did not practice yoga gained about 14 pounds over that 10-year period.

Why does yoga work so well for fighting fat? The researchers suspected that it has to do with increased body awareness rather than the physical activity itself— in other words, a better appreciation of one's body, stress relief, an enhanced awareness of satiety, and not wanting to overeat. Yoga is clearly powerful stuff.

Although there have not been studies like this done on Pilates, tai chi, or qigong, I believe that they would work the same way, since these activities relieve stress, relax your body and mind, and help you be extra loving to yourself.

Lifestyle activities. I am adding a fourth bucket here—lifestyle activities. What I mean is simply moving around—walking upstairs, playing with your kids, gardening, biking, doing household chores, sitting less, and so forth. These things are not exercise; they are movement. Moving the way humans have moved as long as we've existed helps to lower your setpoint, because they are the way we were designed to move. The more you move naturally like this, the more enjoyable your life will be. Plus, if you want to be able to move later in life, it's a good idea to move earlier in life.

THE SANE MIND-SET

At the core of the SANE mind-set is loving yourself for who you are and recognizing that forces in the world have created a warped, unrealistic image of the way people should look. The psychological tools you now have are designed to give you self-nurturing, self-compassionate ways to treat yourself—and to see that you are worth it and that you are truly beautiful, inside and out. Once you love yourself fully, you will be forever free from the overeating or self-destructive lifestyle choices caused by shame and guilt.

Remember, SANE has not been a quick fix. It has required a lot of smart work on your part. It's not possible, nor is it realistic, to instantly love yourself, change your bad habits, and get on with life—rather, it's a gradual change.

You started changing your life when you got honest about the diets and gimmicks that failed you in the past. You saw a pattern emerge, and as this pattern became clear, you were filled with genuine hope for what your future held in store. Why? Because this pattern convinced you once and for all, "It really wasn't me that failed; it was all those weight-loss myths that I have been told for years." Your eyes were opened to how horribly the approach of "just eat less" and "exercise more" had let you down, and with that realization your life began to change.

Fast fixes just never work. If they did, they would have worked already. SANE is all about courageous consistency, unconditional self-love, and calm patience. Changing the way you eat, the way you move, the way you think, and the way you live on a consistent, daily basis is the key to lowering your setpoint, which you now know is the *only* way to lose weight permanently. "Going SANE" is not a temporary change; it's a whole new way to approach yourself and your life.

If you read this book and did the plan, then I know you saw results. You are now #SANE4Life. If you say, "Hey, Jonathan, I'm not ready to make that sort of lifelong commitment," that's fine, and may I just ask you to sit with a question overnight. No need to agree or disagree, simply let it sit in your mind overnight:

When you began this journey, did you say, "I want to lose 30 pounds, keep it off briefly, then gain it all back, with some extra pounds for good measure?" Of course not, but that is exactly what happens to most people who lose weight—and exactly what probably happened to you in the past. But never again, thanks to your new information, tools, and skills.

Once you do the plan and see the results, there is no going back to what life was before SANE. You have been transformed inside and out, body and mind. Like the butterfly that emerges from the cocoon, you cannot go back to your previous life, and you can't unknow what you now know. And thanks to your SANE mind-set, you'll never want to because you know that you deserve nothing less than the best.

You have a lot going for you psychologically now. You understand the psychological principle that says what people think about, even fixate on, are the exact things that they are trying to move away from in life, and that very strategy is what causes them to constantly suffer through the exact opposite of what they want.

Take your own life, for example. Have you ever had a hard time falling asleep and then found that the harder you try to fall asleep, the more awake you felt? Or how about the last time you tried not to worry about something? Maybe you needed to speak in public and the more you told yourself, "Calm down…calm down…calm down!" the less and less calm you became? Or how about the times you tried to cut back on sweets? To help you avoid sweets, you told yourself over and over, "Do not eat sweets. Do not even think about sweets." What happened was that you thought about sweets 24/7!

Look at all those failed diets. What did they have in common? In short, no matter what sexy name they had, and no matter how hard they tried to hide it, they all focused on the same thing: what NOT to do.

Modern psychology shows that focusing on what you don't want will cause more of it to show up in your life. You are done with that ineffective approach and are now enjoying a SANEr and more effective path: pursuing the positive (instead of attacking the negative). With this simple switch, you are making your brain work for you rather than against you. You are focused on eating *more* SANE foods. And with that simple mental shift, gue what that monitoring process in your brain focuses on? Where can I find more healing food? How can I enjoy more healing food? And if your subconscious is constantly coming up with so many ways to eat so much delicious SANE food that there just isn't room for any inSANE setpoint-elevating processed nonsense, this fundamentally different approach MUST give you a fundamentally different result. In fact, researchers at Université Laval in Quebec have been studying this mental shift to eating more healing food versus less of everything and found this approach to be almost unbelievably more effective than the "do NOT eat" message you've been fed for years.

You also learned and applied the power of setting small process goals—which are so deeply empowering for your mind-set. Every week, you focused on small process goals, framed by intention implementations, to help you achieve your goals. Keep going! To paraphrase an old proverb, "If you are facing in the right direction, just keep walking and eventually you will get there." That is the power of process goals.

Be sure to keep writing in your gratitude journal. This helps you override negative self-talk and is a proven way to love yourself slim. So is maintaining your involvement in a SANE support group. Studies show that people who abandon the support systems they used to lose weight are much more likely to regain the weight than people who stay in touch.

Throughout our time together, you have been working with your psychology and biology rather than against it. And you finally see the results you have wanted for so long. This fundamentally different approach—SANE living—has given you a fundamentally different result.

As you have discovered throughout this book, the SANE approach is based on proven science and practical engineering, not opinions nor gimmicks. It is not an opinion that your body regulates your weight automatically. Calories do have different qualities. Hormones are important. Starches are more harmful than helpful. Added sweeteners are addictive and toxic. Protein and fat are essential while carbohydrates are not. Non-starchy vegetables, nutrient-dense protein, whole-food fats, and low-fructose fruits are the SANEst foods. They give you the most pure and nutritious fuel possible so that you and everyone you love can live the best life possible. Because you have healed your mind along with your body while eating *more* and exercising *less* than ever, you can easily keep this up long-term.

With the awareness you have gained, you proved to yourself that you have the inner strength to achieve goals, change habits, and improve your life for the better.

You have a beautiful light shining within you. You are shedding everything that has been keeping that light from shining, and you can see a bright future ahead of you full of happiness and limitless possibility. You have the right to feel attractive and healthy, the right to be proud of who you are, the right to be excited about your life, and the right to be treated with respect by others, and nothing is going to stop you now. Not because I say so. But because modern science proves it, and because practical engineering enables it, and because you are living it.

A FINAL FAVOR

You and I have come a long way together, and I know for you the journey is still unfolding, so may I ask for a favor? While this may seem odd initially, please put the following reflection on your refrigerator and desk and read it out loud twice daily (a printable version is available at SANESolution.com). This simple habit will do more for your long-term sanity and SANEity than every disproven "eat less, exercise more" gimmick and quick fix combined. It's called "My SANEity" and it was collaboratively written by some of our most successful members in the SANE program, our most senior SANE Certified Coaches, and myself. It reflects why we've dedicated our lives to restoring SANEity to an insane world, and why we are so grateful you've chosen to join us.

My SANEity

If "just tell me what to eat" worked, I would be "eating it" already.

If counting calories and points worked, I would be "thin" already.

If trying to be perfect worked, I would be "perfect" already.

If quick fixes worked, I would be "fixed" already.

So what works?

Well...What *haven't* I tried yet?

Courageous consistency?

Unconditional self-love?

Calm patience?

SANE eating?

THAT is what works.

To achieve a different result, I will take a different approach.

Living SANE works. It will. It is proven biology.

So I will give myself the courageous consistency, unconditional self-love, calm patience, and proven SANEity I deserve!

And with patient, consistent, and self-loving SANEity, I will permanently enjoy the energy, body, health, and happiness of my dreams! I will be SANE.

I saved this till the very end. It's the big reveal. The "insider's" secret to lifelong slimness, fitness, and health. Ready? The secret, the one thing that once you get it will instantly enable you to achieve everything you want in the world of wellness is this:

The secret is that there is no secret. Eat the most satisfying, hormonally healthy, nutritious, and inefficient natural foods in abundance, while moving your body intelligently, thinking empoweringly, resting frequently, contributing to others daily, and loving deeply. A healthy body, mind, and spirit results in a lower setpoint and so...much...more.

A high-quality life is the result of high-quality living. You are of the highest quality. You and everyone else in your life deserves nothing less than the highest quality. And that's why you are living a life of pursuing the positive (high-quality) rather than attacking the negative (low-quality). You become what you focus on. Focus on higher quality and everything in your world—especially yourself—becomes higher quality.

So as we wrap up, I hope that you are filled with hope and fully empowered because you have concretely proven to yourself that you haven't failed. You aren't broken. In fact, just the opposite is true. You now have a way of life that finally gives you what you've longed for in terms of leanness, better health, and self-worth.

Here's to a lifetime of enjoying a lower setpoint and being naturally thin, transformed, and fulfilled—the even more beautiful new you. Here's to the highest-quality life imaginable. Here's to your SANEity.

ACKNOWLEDGMENTS

This book is the result of more than fifteen years of collaboration with thousands of brilliant and inspiring researchers and SANE Family Members. To everyone who helped bring this proven science and powerful love to the surface: I cannot thank you enough for your time, insight, and support. Together we will make the world a SANEr place.

To Wednesday Vail, Tyler Archer, Maggie Robinson, and Jodi Lipper, this book exists because of you. Thank you for bringing these lifesaving words to life. To Celeste Fine, Sarah Passick, and Anna Petkovich at Sterling Lord Literistic, you have so far transcended the traditional literary agent role, and I am in awe. Thank you for making my dreams come true. Thank you to the tremendous team at Hachette Book Group and beyond for facilitating this once-in-a-lifetime opportunity. To my executive editors, Amanda Murray and Michelle Howry, your passion and commitment to this project were obvious and inspiring from day one. Thank you for your unwavering support and trust and for the immeasurable value you added to this project. You exceeded expectations every step of the way. To CiCi Cunningham, none of this would be possible without your championing, insights, and generosity. To marketing geniuses Michael Barrs and Odette Fleming, my publicist Anna Hall, my publishers Mauro DiPreta and Michelle Aielli, assistants Mollie Weisenfeld and Lauren Hummel, and art director Amanda Kain: Proven science, practical habits, and powerful love are only as helpful as they are available to the public. Thank you for the passion and creativity you bring to making this lifesaving research accessible to everyone.

Thank you to the most incredible person I have ever met in my life: my best friend, my partner, my everything, my beloved, my wife, Angela. Every day I'm met with wonderment as to how lucky I am to spend my life and my forever with such an angelic being. This book and the broader dream it reflects would not exist were it not for your remarkable support and collaboration.

Thank you to my family. Robert, Mary-Rose, Tim, Patty, Terry, Carolyn,

Scott, Cameron, and Branden. You are such treasures. Thank you for being who you are and thank you for meaning so much to me.

Thank you to the dazzling SANE Family and Team. You are why I wake up. You are my purpose. Thank you for your trust and for being #SANE4Life. I promise to earn it.

Thank you to my enlightened mentors and business partners, Joshua Pokempner and Jason Anderson. You are angels in every sense of the word. Thank you for giving so much of yourselves to such a noble mission.

Finally, thank you to every member of SANE movement worldwide. The support you have shown from day one has consistently caused me to get teary-eyed. You have the courage to replace starvation, shame, and stress with proven science, practical habits, and powerful love. You have taken the road less traveled and it will make all the difference.

APPENDIX A

SANE Setpoint-Lowering Recipes

EGG DISHES

Mom's Favorite Frittata

Yield: 2
Total Time: 40 minutes
Prep: 10 minutes • **Cook:** 30 minutes

1–2 teaspoons extra-virgin coconut oil (enough to lightly coat your
  pan when hot)
½ red onion, finely chopped
1 red bell pepper, seeded and chopped
1 jalapeño pepper, minced (remove ribs and seeds for less spiciness)
4 eggs and 12 egg whites
¼ cup Parmesan cheese, grated (optional)
½ teaspoon Tabasco sauce
½ teaspoon salt
½ teaspoon dried oregano
¼ teaspoon ground black pepper

- Preheat oven to 350°F.
- Melt most of the coconut oil in a large frying pan set over medium heat. Add the onion and cook, stirring often, for 2 minutes. Add the red pepper and jalapeño and cook for 2 more minutes. Remove from heat.
- In a large bowl, whisk the eggs. Stir in the cheese, Tabasco, seasonings, and the onion mixture.
- Generously oil a 9-inch pie plate with remaining oil.
- Whisk the egg mixture again, pour into the pie plate, and bake in the center of the oven until the top is golden, 25–30 minutes. Serve hot or at room temperature.

SANE Scoring: Each serving of this recipe supplies non-starchy vegetables (1 serving), nutrient-dense protein (1 serving, 30 grams), whole-food fats (1 serving).

Kale Marinara

Yield: 2
Total Time: 13 minutes
Prep: 5 minutes • **Cook:** 8 minutes

Garlic clove, chopped
½ medium onion, chopped
1–2 teaspoons extra-virgin coconut oil (enough to lightly coat your
    pan when hot)
8 ounces of extra-lean ground beef
1 to 1½ cups all-natural no sugar added pasta sauce
2 eggs
Baby kale leaves, 2 handfuls
Salt, to taste

- Sauté garlic and onion in extra-virgin coconut oil. Add in meat and cook for a few minutes. Add in pasta sauce and cook down for 5 minutes.
- Scramble eggs in a different pan and add into pasta sauce. Add in the kale leaves last and cook until wilted. Salt and serve.

SANE Scoring: Each serving of this recipe supplies non-starchy vegetables (1 serving), nutrient-dense protein (1 serving, 30 grams), and whole-food fats (1 serving).

Denver Scrambled Eggs

Yield: 1
Total Time: 20 minutes
Prep: 5 minutes • **Cook:** 15 minutes

1–2 teaspoons extra-virgin coconut oil (enough to lightly coat your
    pan when hot)
⅓ cup white onions, chopped
½ cup green bell pepper, chopped

1 small whole red tomato, diced
⅛ teaspoon red or cayenne pepper
Salt and freshly ground pepper, to taste
2 large eggs (whole)
4 ounces boneless, cooked fresh ham

- Heat oil in large heavy skillet over medium heat. Sauté onion 5 minutes, until softened. Add green peppers, tomatoes, and red or cayenne pepper. Cover and cook 5 minutes, until vegetables are very soft, stirring occasionally. Season with salt and pepper and set aside.
- In small bowl, beat eggs until blended. Set aside.
- In large nonstick skillet, add the ham and cook 3 minutes or until it just begins to brown on the edges. Add the pepper mixture and then the eggs. Stir the mixture until the eggs begin to scramble, about 5 minutes. Serve immediately.

SANE Scoring: Each serving of this recipe supplies non-starchy vegetables (1 serving), nutrient-dense protein (1 serving, 37 grams), and whole-food fats (1 serving).

CHICKEN AND TURKEY RECIPES

Breakfast Meatloaf

Yield: 8
Total Time: 1 hour 10 minutes
Prep: 15 minutes • **Cook:** 55 minutes

16 ounces frozen spinach, chopped and thawed
4 medium stalks of celery, diced
2 medium red bell peppers, chopped
2 medium green bell peppers, chopped
1 small onion, chopped
1½ pounds of turkey breakfast sausage
1½ pounds of lean ground turkey
6 large eggs (whole)
½ teaspoon ground dried thyme
⅛ teaspoon ground nutmeg
⅛ teaspoon red or cayenne pepper

½ teaspoon of garlic powder (optional)
Salt and freshly ground pepper, to taste

- Preheat oven to 350°F.
- Combine the vegetables with the ground turkey sausage and turkey, and mix thoroughly. Add the eggs and spices. Distribute evenly and place in two standard quick bread pans (4×9 inches).
- Bake until cooked through and browned on top, about 55–65 minutes. Serve immediately or freeze in individual portions for up to 2 months.

SANE Scoring: Each serving of this recipe supplies non-starchy vegetables (1 serving), nutrient-dense protein (1 serving, 40 grams), and whole-food fats (1 serving).

Turkey Stuffed Peppers

Yield: 8
Total Time: 50 minutes
Prep: 20 minutes • **Cook:** 30 minutes

8 green bell peppers, tops and seeds removed
2 pounds extra-lean ground turkey
1–2 teaspoons extra-virgin coconut oil (enough to lightly coat your pan when hot)
1 onion, chopped finely
2 cups sliced mushrooms
2 zucchini, chopped
1 red bell pepper, chopped
1 yellow bell pepper, chopped
2 cups fresh spinach
2 (14.5 ounce) cans diced tomatoes, drained
2 tablespoons tomato paste
Italian seasoning, to taste (about 1 tablespoon)
Garlic powder, to taste (about ½ to 1 teaspoon)
Salt and freshly ground pepper, to taste

- Preheat oven to 350°F.
- Wrap the green bell peppers in aluminum foil, and place in a baking dish. Bake for 15 minutes.
- While the green peppers are baking, cook the ground turkey until browned in a skillet over medium heat. Set cooked turkey aside. Heat the coconut oil in the skillet, and cook the onions, mushrooms, zucchini, red and yellow peppers, and spinach until softened. Add the turkey back into the skillet. Mix in the

tomatoes, tomato paste, and seasonings. Fill the green peppers with the skillet mixture.

- Return the now stuffed peppers to the oven, and cook another 15 minutes.

SANE Scoring: Each serving of this recipe supplies non-starchy vegetables (3 servings), nutrient-dense protein (1 serving, 26 grams).

Italian Chicken Skillet

Yield: 8
Total Time: 40 minutes
Prep: 20 minutes • **Cook:** 20 minutes

1½ cups chicken broth
3 tablespoons tomato paste
½ teaspoon freshly ground black pepper
1 teaspoon dried oregano
¼ teaspoon salt
2 cloves garlic, minced
8 boneless, skinless chicken breast halves
¼ cup and 2 tablespoons almond meal
1 tablespoon extra-virgin coconut oil
4 cups fresh sliced mushrooms

- In a medium bowl, combine the broth, tomato paste, ground black pepper, oregano, salt, and garlic. Mix well and set aside.
- Dredge the chicken in the almond meal, coating well. Heat the oil in a large skillet over medium-high heat. Sauté the chicken in the oil for 2 minutes per side, or until lightly browned. Add the reserved broth mixture and the mushrooms to the skillet and bring to a boil. Then cover, reduce heat to low, and simmer for 20 minutes. Remove chicken and set aside, covering to keep it warm.
- Bring the broth mixture to a boil and cook for 4 minutes, or until reduced to desired thickness. Spoon sauce over the chicken and serve.

SANE Scoring: Each serving of this recipe supplies nutrient-dense protein (1 serving, 30 grams) and whole-food fats (1 serving).

Balsamic Chicken

Yield: 8
Total Time: 25 minutes
Prep: 5 minutes • **Cook:** 20 minutes

⅔ cup balsamic vinegar
1 cup chicken broth
¼ cup xylitol or erythritol (both optional)
2 cloves garlic, minced
2 teaspoons dried Italian herb seasoning
8 skinless, boneless chicken breast halves
1–2 teaspoons extra-virgin coconut oil (enough to lightly coat your
     pan when hot)

- Whisk together the balsamic vinegar, chicken broth, xylitol, garlic, and Italian seasoning in a bowl to create a marinade. Place the chicken breasts in the marinade, and marinate for 10 minutes on each side.
- Heat the extra-virgin coconut oil in a large skillet over medium-high heat. Remove the chicken from the marinade and reserve the marinade. Place the chicken breast halves in the heated pan and cook until they start to brown and are no longer pink inside, about 7 minutes per side. Pour the marinade into the skillet, bringing it to a full rolling boil, and cook until it thickens slightly, turning the chicken breasts over once or twice, about 5 minutes.

SANE Scoring: Each serving of this recipe supplies nutrient-dense protein (1 serving, 30 grams).

Tex-Mex Chicken

Yield: 8
Total Time: 40 minutes
Prep: 15 minutes • **Cook:** 25 minutes

Coconut oil cooking spray
8 skinless, boneless chicken breasts
2 cloves garlic, minced
2 pinches salt
2 pinches ground black pepper
2 pinches ground cumin

2 cups salsa
2 cups shredded cheddar cheese

- Preheat oven to 375°F.
- Coat a skillet with cooking spray and heat to medium. Rub chicken pieces with garlic, salt, pepper, and cumin to taste; place in the hot skillet. Cook until brown on both sides and no longer pink, 10–15 minutes.
- Transfer chicken to 9×13-inch baking dish or casserole dish, top with salsa and cheese, and bake in preheated oven until cheese is bubbly and starts to brown, about 15–20 minutes.

SANE Scoring: Each serving of this recipe supplies nutrient-dense protein (1 serving, 40 grams) and dairy (1 serving).

PORK RECIPES

Garlic Herb Pork

Yield: 5
Total Time: 50 minutes
Prep: 5 minutes • **Cook:** 45 minutes

1½ to 2 pounds boneless roast pork
4 garlic cloves, peeled and crushed
2 teaspoons coarse salt
1 tablespoon fresh sage, minced
2 teaspoons fresh rosemary, minced
¼ teaspoon black pepper
1 tablespoon extra-virgin coconut oil

- Preheat oven to 450°F.
- Pat pork dry with paper towel and place in shallow roasting pan.
- In a small bowl, mix all the remaining ingredients together and rub all over the pork.
- Place pork in oven and roast for 15 minutes. Lower temperature to 300°F and roast another 20 minutes or until pork reaches 150°F on thermometer.
- Remove pork and let rest for 5 minutes, covered loosely with a tent of aluminum foil.

SANE Scoring: Each serving of this recipe supplies nutrient-dense protein (1 serving, 38–51 grams) and whole-food fats (1 serving).

Lemon-Garlic Pork Kebabs

Yield: 8
Total Time: 30 minutes
Prep: 15 minutes • **Cook:** 15 minutes

Pork
> 2 pounds boneless pork tenderloin, cut in 1 ½-inch cubes
> Extra-virgin coconut oil

Marinade
> ⅓ cup lemon juice
> 1 tablespoon garlic, minced
> ½ teaspoon dried rosemary

- Mix marinade ingredients in a plastic zipper bag. Add pork cubes and marinate at least 1 hour but not more than 6.
- Thread meat on skewers. Brush with extra-virgin coconut oil. Grill or broil on medium-low heat for 7–10 minutes on each side or until nicely browned and just barely done. Don't overcook or they will be dry and tough.

SANE Scoring: Each serving of this recipe supplies nutrient-dense protein (1 serving, 30 grams).

Slow Cooker Pulled Pork

Yield: 8
Total Time: 6–8 hours
Prep: 20 minutes • **Cook:** 6–8 hours

> 5 cloves of garlic, peeled
> 1 large onion, quartered
> 1½ tablespoons fresh oregano
> 1½ tablespoons ground cumin
> 1 tablespoon ground ancho chili pepper
> 3 teaspoons salt
> 3 teaspoons freshly ground black pepper
> 1½ tablespoons white wine vinegar
> 1 (3-pound) boneless pork sirloin tip roast
> 1 lime, cut into wedges

- Put all the ingredients, except the lime wedges, into the slow cooker. Cook on low until the pork is fork tender, 6–8 hours. Remove the pork.

- Blend everything left in the pot (an immersion blender is helpful here). Return the pork to the pot and shred into the sauce. Garnish with lime wedges to serve.

SANE Scoring: Each serving of this recipe supplies nutrient-dense protein (1 serving, 37 grams).

BEEF DISHES

Asian Marinated Flank Steak

Yield: 4
Total Time: 30–40 minutes
Prep: 10 minutes • **Cook:** 20–30 minutes

¼ cup water
¼ cup soy sauce
2 tablespoons rice vinegar
2 tablespoons ginger root, grated
1 pinch chili flakes
2 pounds flank steak

- Place all ingredients except for steak in a gallon-sized zip-top bag, and mix well to combine. Add steak to bag. Remove all of the air, and seal. Marinate for up to 24 hours, turning bag occasionally.
- Remove meat from marinade, and grill or broil to desired degree of doneness. Thinly slice steak against the grain and serve.
- You can substitute (or add) garlic for the ginger. If you like it spicy, add more chili flakes!

SANE Scoring: Each serving of this recipe supplies nutrient-dense protein (1 serving, 40 grams).

Braised Beef

Yield: 6
Total Time: 1 hour 10 minutes
Prep: 10 minutes • **Cook:** 1 hour

2 pounds round steaks, cut ½-inch thick
3 slices uncooked bacon
1 cup water

¼ cup carrot, chopped
¼ cup celery, chopped
2 tablespoons fresh parsley, chopped
1 medium bay leaf
1–2 teaspoons extra-virgin coconut oil (enough to lightly coat your
    pan when hot)
1 tablespoon onion, chopped
¼ cup mushrooms, chopped
¼ cup nonfat Greek yogurt
2 tablespoons capers

- Cut steak in serving-sized pieces.
- Cook bacon in a large skillet until crisp; remove, crumble, and set aside.
- Brown steak in bacon drippings. Add water, carrot, celery, and bay leaf; cover
  and cook over low heat 1½ hours, or until meat is tender, stirring occasionally.
  Remove bay leaf and remove beef to a serving platter and keep warm.
- Meanwhile, in a separate skillet, melt coconut oil over medium-low heat. Add
  onions and mushrooms and sauté until tender, about 5 minutes. Add to first
  skillet and blend with an immersion blender or process in a stand-up blender.
  Stir in yogurt and capers; heat through. Pour gravy over steaks; garnish with
  bacon crumbles and chopped parsley.

*SANE Scoring: Each serving of this recipe supplies nutrient-dense protein (1 serving, 30 grams)
and whole-food fats (1 serving).*

Slow Cooker Fiesta Beef

Yield: 8
Total Time: 11 hours 15 minutes
Prep: 15 minutes • **Cook:** 11 hours

4 pounds beef chuck roast, trimmed of fat and meat cut into chunks
1 (24-ounce) jar salsa
1 medium onion, chopped
1 (7-ounce) can chopped mild green chilis
2 cloves garlic, minced
2 teaspoons chili powder
1 ½ teaspoons ground cumin
½ teaspoon dried oregano

- Place chuck roast, salsa, onion, green chile peppers, garlic, chili powder, cumin, and oregano in a slow cooker. Cook on low for 10–12 hours. Remove lid and cook on high for 1 more hour.
- Remove chuck roast from slow cooker using a slotted spoon and transfer it to a serving platter; shred meat with a fork. Add liquid from slow cooker, 1 tablespoon at a time, to the chuck roast until desired consistency is reached.

SANE Scoring: Each serving of this recipe supplies nutrient-dense protein (1 serving, 54 grams) and whole-food fats (2 servings).

Slow Cooker Tomato & Herb Beef

Yield: 8
Total Time: 8 hours 20 min
Prep: 20 minutes • **Cook:** 8 hours

1 (3-pound) boneless bottom round roast, trimmed of fat
Freshly ground pepper, to taste
1 tablespoon extra-virgin coconut oil
1 medium onion, thinly sliced
1 medium carrot, shredded
2 garlic cloves, minced (or pressed)
2 teaspoons dried Italian herb seasoning
1 (15-ounce) can tomato sauce
1 tablespoon Worcestershire sauce
¼ cup dry red wine
Chopped parsley

- Sprinkle pepper on all sides of beef. Heat oil in a wide nonstick frying pan over medium-high heat; add beef and brown well on all sides.
- Meanwhile, in a 3-quart or larger electric slow cooker, combine onion, carrot, garlic, and herb seasoning.
- In a small bowl, mix tomato sauce, Worcestershire, and wine; set aside.
- Place beef on top of onion mixture. Pour tomato sauce mixture over beef. Cover and cook at low setting until beef is very tender when pierced (8–10 hours).
- Lift beef to a warm platter and keep warm. Skim and discard fat from sauce, if necessary. To serve, slice beef across the grain. Spoon some of the sauce over meat; garnish with parsley. Serve remaining sauce separately.

SANE Scoring: Each serving of this recipe supplies nutrient-dense protein (1 serving, 50 grams) and whole-food fats (1 serving).

Marinated Sirloin

Yield: 8
Total Time: 15 minutes
Prep: 5 minutes • **Cook:** 10 minutes

2 tablespoons extra-virgin coconut oil
¼ cup onion, minced
2 tablespoons lemon juice
2 tablespoons Worcestershire sauce
2 tablespoons soy sauce
2 teaspoons garlic powder
1 teaspoon freshly ground black pepper
3 pounds sirloin steak

- Whisk together melted coconut oil, onion, lemon juice, Worcestershire sauce, soy sauce, garlic powder, and pepper in a bowl until marinade is well mixed. Place steak in a large resealable plastic bag and pour marinade over meat. Coat meat with marinade, squeeze out excess air, and seal bag. Marinate in the refrigerator for at least 4 hours, turning occasionally.
- Preheat grill for medium heat and lightly oil the grate. Drain steak and discard marinade. Cook steaks on the preheated grill until they are beginning to firm and are hot and slightly pink in the center, 5 minutes per side. An instant-read thermometer inserted into the center should read 140°F.

SANE Scoring: Each serving of this recipe supplies nutrient-dense protein (2 servings, 37 grams) and whole-food fats (2 servings).

FISH RECIPES

Canned Tuna Ceviche

Yield: 2
Total Time: 15 minutes
Prep: 15 minutes

2 (7-ounce) cans of tuna
1 fresh jalapeño chile, seeded and minced (more or less, to taste)
1 small red onion, peeled and finely chopped

1 ripe tomato, diced
1 tablespoon fresh cilantro, chopped
Salt, to taste
Freshly ground black pepper, to taste
¼ cup fresh lime juice (1–2 limes)
1 avocado, diced or mashed
Lettuce leaves, 2
Fresh cilantro stem, for garnish

- Drain the tuna and invert it onto a small platter. Sprinkle the chile and onion over the tuna and allow it to stand for a few minutes. Then add the tomato, chopped cilantro, diced avocado, and salt and pepper to taste, and gently mix together.
- Sprinkle the lime juice over all. Serve over lettuce if you like. Garnish with sprigs of cilantro and serve.

SANE Scoring: Each serving of this recipe supplies nutrient-dense protein (1 serving, 50 grams) and whole-food fats (1 serving).

Dijon Salmon

Yield: 8
Total Time: 35 minutes
Prep: 15 minutes • **Cook:** 20 minutes

Coconut oil cooking spray
8 (6-ounce) salmon fillets
⅔ cup Dijon mustard
4 large garlic cloves, thinly sliced
2 red onions, thinly sliced
2 teaspoons dried tarragon
Salt and pepper, to taste

- Preheat oven to 400°F. Spray a 9×13-inch pan with coconut oil cooking spray.
- Arrange the salmon skin side down in the prepared pan, and lightly coat with the Dijon mustard. Place the garlic and onion slices on the salmon fillets. Season with tarragon, salt, and pepper.
- Bake 20 minutes in the preheated oven, or until salmon is easily flaked with a fork.

SANE Scoring: Each serving of this recipe supplies nutrient-dense protein (1 serving, 45 grams) and whole-food fats (2 servings).

Tuna Teriyaki

Yield: 8
Total Time: 25 minutes
Prep: 15 minutes • **Cook:** 10 minutes

2 cups no-sugar teriyaki sauce
1 tablespoon extra-virgin coconut oil
¼ cup garlic, minced
2 teaspoons freshly ground black pepper
8 (4-ounce) fillets yellowfin tuna

- In a large resealable plastic bag, combine the teriyaki sauce, oil, garlic, and pepper. Place the tuna fillets in the bag. Seal the bag with as little air in it as possible. Give the mix a good shake to ensure the tuna fillets are well coated. Marinate for 30 minutes in the refrigerator.
- Meanwhile, preheat an outdoor grill for high heat, and lightly oil grate.
- Remove tuna from marinade, and place on grill. For rare tuna, grill for 3–5 minutes on each side. For medium tuna, grill 5–8 minutes per side. For well-done tuna, grill for 8–10 minutes per side.

SANE Scoring: Each serving of this recipe supplies nutrient-dense protein (2 servings, 27 grams).

Bayou Shrimp

Yield: 8
Total Time: 10 minutes
Prep: 5 minutes • **Cook:** 5 minutes

2 teaspoons paprika
1½ teaspoons dried thyme
1½ teaspoons dried oregano
½ teaspoon garlic powder
½ teaspoon salt
½ teaspoon ground black pepper
½ teaspoon cayenne pepper, or more, to taste
3 pounds large shrimp, peeled and deveined
1–2 teaspoons extra-virgin coconut oil (enough to lightly coat your
    pan when hot)

- Combine paprika, thyme, oregano, garlic powder, salt, pepper, and cayenne pepper in a sealable plastic bag; shake to mix. Add shrimp and shake to coat.
- Heat oil in a large nonstick skillet over medium-high heat. Cook and stir shrimp in hot oil until they are bright pink on the outside and the meat is no longer transparent in the center, about 4 minutes.

SANE Scoring: Each serving of this recipe supplies nutrient-dense protein (1 serving, 35 grams).

PLANT-BASED MAIN DISHES

Mushroom Tofu Scramble

Yield: 4
Total Time: 16 minutes
Prep: 10 minutes • **Cook:** 6 minutes

1 cup white onions, chopped
4 cups mushrooms, chopped
2 tablespoons extra-virgin coconut oil
2 (14-ounce) packages extra-firm lite tofu
4 cups baby spinach
4 eggs and 12 egg whites
¼ cup Parmesan cheese, grated (or substitute 2 tablespoons
      nutritional yeast)
⅛ teaspoon dried thyme
8 cherry tomatoes

- In a large nonstick skillet cook the onions and mushrooms in the coconut oil over medium-high heat, until soft (about 3 minutes). Add the tofu and spinach, and cook an additional 3 minutes. Stir in the tomatoes, eggs, egg whites, cheese, and thyme and cook until the eggs are firm.
- Serve immediately.

SANE Scoring: Each serving of this recipe supplies non-starchy vegetables (2 servings), nutrient-dense protein (1 serving, 43 grams), and whole-food fats (1 serving).

Simple Baked Tofu

Yield: 2
Total Time: 50 minutes
Prep: 20 minutes • **Cook:** 30 minutes

2 (14-ounce) packages firm tofu
¼ cup soy sauce
2 tablespoons rice vinegar
1 tablespoon extra-virgin coconut oil

- Preheat oven to 350°F.
- Wrap the tofu in paper towels and press under a heavy skillet for 15 minutes. If it's still pretty wet, replace the towels and press it again.
- Mix the soy sauce, vinegar, and oil in a container that is small but big enough for all the tofu.
- Cut the tofu in ½-inch slices and place in marinade. Turn it over after about 15 minutes. Wipe some of the oil from the marinade on your baking sheet.
- Arrange the tofu slices in one layer and bake for 15 minutes. Turn them over and bake another 15 minutes.

SANE Scoring: Each serving of this recipe supplies nutrient-dense protein (1 serving, 32 grams).

Asian Tofu

Yield: 4
Total Time: 1 hour 15 minutes
Prep: 30 minutes • **Cook:** 45 minutes

4 (12-ounce) packages firm lite tofu
1 tablespoon extra-virgin coconut oil
¼ cup soy sauce
2 tablespoons rice wine
2 tablespoons rice vinegar
2 garlic cloves, minced
¼ cup onions, finely minced
2 teaspoons grated fresh ginger
¼ cup water
1 teaspoon hot chili paste, to taste (optional)

- Preheat oven to 375°F.
- For best results, tofu should be "pressed" in order to remove excess liquid and absorb the flavors of the marinade. Press tofu block between two plates, weighted down with a cast-iron pan, large bowl of water, or heavy cans, for about 30 minutes. Halfway through, you may remove the plate of water and flip the tofu block. After tofu is pressed, cut the block into small cubes or triangles.
- Whisk together the ingredients in a bowl.
- Place pieces of tofu into baking dish, and cover with the marinade. The tofu can sit overnight in the marinade or can be prepared right away. Bake tofu about 35–45 minutes, or until all the liquid is absorbed.

SANE Scoring: Each serving of this recipe supplies nutrient-dense protein (1 serving, 32 grams).

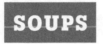

Broccoli Soup

Yield: 6
Total Time: 35 minutes
Prep: 15 minutes • **Cook:** 20 minutes

5 cups broccoli, diced
2 cups carrots, sliced
½ cup onion, chopped
6 cups water
1 teaspoon dried oregano
1 teaspoon dried basil
4 chicken bouillon cubes or 4 tablespoons chicken bouillon powder
    (or you can substitute chicken stock for the water)
Salt and pepper, to taste

- In a 5-quart saucepan, add all ingredients except salt and pepper. Cover and simmer until vegetables are tender (about 20 minutes).
- Strain off and reserve most of the liquid. Place vegetables in a food processor and puree. Add pureed vegetables and reserved liquid (if you wish for a more liquid soup) back into the pot. Add salt and pepper and reheat.

SANE Scoring: Each serving of this recipe supplies non-starchy vegetables (1 serving).

Cream of Cauliflower Soup

Yield: 6
Total Time: 1 hour 5 minutes
Prep: 5 minutes • **Cook:** 1 hour

1 medium head cauliflower, cut into florets
2 stalks celery, cut into pieces
1 medium onion, chopped
Salt and pepper, to taste
4–6 cups chicken broth
½ cup coconut cream (optional)
½ teaspoon Worcestershire sauce
⅛ teaspoon nutmeg

- In a big stock pot, add broth, cauliflower, celery, onion, salt, and pepper. Cook until tender, about 1 hour or until cool.
- Blend the mixture in a blender until smooth. Pour back into pot; add Worcestershire sauce, nutmeg, and coconut cream. Cook until soup is ready to boil.

SANE Scoring: Each serving of this recipe supplies non-starchy vegetables (1 serving).

Ginger Carrot Soup

Yield: 4
Total Time: 40 minutes
Prep: 15 minutes • **Cook:** 25 minutes

8 carrots (1 pound), sliced, leaves reserved for garnish
1 tablespoon fresh ginger, chopped
1 large clove garlic, smashed
¼ teaspoon crushed red pepper, plus additional for garnish
½ teaspoon kosher salt
4 cups water
2 teaspoons fresh lemon juice

- In large pot, simmer all ingredients except lemon juice in water until carrots are tender (20–25 minutes).
- Using an immersion blender (or a standard blender working in batches), blend until smooth; add lemon juice. Divide among 4 bowls; garnish with crushed red pepper and carrot leaves. If desired, serve chilled.

SANE Scoring: Each serving of this recipe supplies non-starchy vegetables (1 serving).

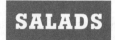

Asparagus Spring Salad

Yield: 12
Total Time: 25 minutes
Prep: 20 minutes • **Cook:** 5 minutes

2 tablespoons rice vinegar
2 teaspoons red wine vinegar
2 teaspoons soy sauce
2 teaspoons Dijon mustard
⅓ cup extra-virgin olive oil
3 pounds fresh asparagus, trimmed and cut into 2-inch pieces
2 tablespoons sesame seeds

- In a small bowl, whisk together the rice vinegar, red wine vinegar, soy sauce, and mustard. Drizzle in the olive oil while whisking vigorously to emulsify. Set aside.
- Bring a pot of lightly salted water to a boil. Add the asparagus to the water, and cook 3–5 minutes until just tender, but still mostly firm. Remove and rinse under cold water to stop from cooking any further.
- Place the asparagus in a large bowl and drizzle the dressing over it. Toss until evenly coated. Sprinkle with sesame seeds to serve.

SANE Scoring: Each serving of this recipe supplies non-starchy vegetables (1 serving).

Invigorating Thai Cabbage Slaw

Yield: 8
Total Time: 5 minutes
Prep: 5 minutes

3 tablespoons fresh lime juice
3 tablespoons unseasoned rice vinegar
2 tablespoons fish sauce
1 tablespoon water
1 tablespoon creamy peanut butter (or almond butter)
1 teaspoon chili paste with garlic
1 garlic clove, minced
6 cups shredded Napa (Chinese) cabbage
2 cups shredded red cabbage
1 cup red bell pepper strips
1 cup shredded carrot
2 tablespoons chopped dry-roasted peanuts or almonds
1 tablespoon chopped fresh cilantro
1 tablespoon chopped fresh mint

- Combine first 7 ingredients in a large bowl, stirring with a whisk until blended.
- Add cabbages, bell pepper, and carrot, and toss gently to coat. Cover and marinate in refrigerator 1 hour. Stir in the peanuts, cilantro, and mint just before serving.

SANE Scoring: Each serving of this recipe supplies non-starchy vegetables (1 serving).

Spring Arugula Salad

Yield: 12
Total Time: 10 minutes
Prep: 10 minutes

1½ shallots, finely diced
2¼ teaspoons SANE honey (see below)
1½ teaspoons Dijon mustard
¼ teaspoon salt
¼ cup extra-virgin olive oil
Fresh lemon juice, to taste

3 tablespoons unseasoned rice vinegar
12 cherry tomatoes
24 cups arugula

- Combine the shallot, SANE honey, mustard, salt, oil, lemon juice, and vinegar in a jar with a lid. Cover the jar with its lid and shake until the dressing comes together.
- Put the arugula in a large bowl and drizzle dressing over it. Toss to coat, and top with cherry tomatoes.

SANE Scoring: Each serving of this recipe supplies non-starchy vegetables (1 serving).

VEGETABLE SIDES

Baby Carrots Parmesan

Yield: 12
Total Time: 25 minutes
Prep: 5 minutes • **Cook:** 20 minutes

2 pounds baby carrots, chopped
1 tablespoon butter or extra-virgin coconut oil
½ cup Parmesan cheese, grated

- Place carrots into a large pot and cover with water. Bring to a boil over high heat, then reduce heat to medium-low, cover, and simmer until tender, about 15 minutes. Drain.
- Melt butter in a skillet over medium heat. Stir in carrots; cook and stir for 1–2 minutes.
- Sprinkle Parmesan cheese on top. Wait 30 seconds before stirring into carrots. Cook and stir for 2 more minutes.

SANE Scoring: Each serving of this recipe supplies non-starchy vegetables (1 serving).

Green Beans Almondine

Yield: 2
Total Time: 25 minutes
Prep: 5 minutes • **Cook:** 20 minutes

1 pound fresh green beans, rinsed and trimmed
1 tablespoon solid extra-virgin coconut oil
2 tablespoons sliced almonds
Pinch of salt (optional)

- Place green beans in a steamer over 1 inch of boiling water. Cover and cook until tender but still firm, about 10 minutes; drain.
- Meanwhile, melt oil in a skillet over medium heat. Sauté almonds until lightly browned. Season with salt if desired. Stir in green beans, and toss to coat.

SANE Scoring: Each serving of this recipe supplies non-starchy vegetables (3 servings) and whole-food fats (1 serving).

Buffalo Hot Wings Cauliflower

Yield: 4
Total Time: 55 minutes
Prep: 10 minutes • **Cook:** 45 minutes

1 head large (6–7-inch diameter) cauliflower
Coconut oil spray
1 tablespoon extra-virgin coconut oil
4 tablespoons red-hot buffalo wing sauce
3 teaspoons Sriracha hot chili sauce
1 ounce blue or Roquefort cheese

- Preheat oven to 375°F.
- Cut cauliflower into smaller florets and slightly spray with coconut oil. Roast on a baking sheet for 35–40 minutes or until tender.
- While cauliflower is roasting, put hot wing sauce and Sriracha into a small saucepan and heat until boiling. Lower heat and simmer for 10 minutes. Add 1 tablespoon oil, stir until melted, and allow to cool to room temperature. Heat a large sauté pan with remaining oil. Add the cauliflower and sauté until heated through; add the hot sauce and continue to cook for 1 minute, tossing continuously until fully coated. Serve immediately with blue cheese sprinkled on top.

SANE Scoring: Each serving of this recipe supplies non-starchy vegetables (1 serving).

Butter Dill Squash

Yield: 12
Total Time: 25 minutes
Prep: 5 minutes • **Cook:** 20 minutes

4 sliced zucchini
4 sliced yellow squash
½ cup butter
Salt and pepper, to taste
1 tablespoon and 1 teaspoon dried dill weed
2 tablespoons lemon juice

- Put the sliced squashes into a large skillet or saucepan with the butter. Sauté over medium-low heat for 10 minutes. Then add the seasonings.
- Sauté another 10 minutes before adding lemon juice. Serve.

SANE Scoring: Each serving of this recipe supplies non-starchy vegetables (1 serving) and whole-food fats (1 serving).

Cajun Asparagus

Yield: 12
Total Time: 15 minutes
Prep: 5 minutes • **Cook:** 10 minutes

Coconut oil spray
4 pounds asparagus
1 tablespoon and 1 teaspoon Cajun seasoning

- Preheat oven to 425°F.
- Snap the asparagus at the tender part of the stalk. Arrange spears in one layer on a baking sheet. Spray lightly with coconut oil spray; sprinkle with the Cajun seasoning.
- Bake in the preheated oven until tender, about 10 minutes.

SANE Scoring: Each serving of this recipe supplies non-starchy vegetables (1 serving).

DESSERTS

Chocolate Almond Butter Mousse

Yield: 8
Total Time: 5 minutes
Prep: 5 minutes

1 cup natural almond butter
2 cups cocoa powder
⅓ cup erythritol
1 teaspoon vanilla bean powder
1 teaspoon cinnamon
Water as needed

- Place almond butter in a large mixing bowl and microwave for 30 seconds until softened.
- Add the remaining ingredients and mix well. Add water and erythritol as needed for desired consistency and sweetness.

SANE Scoring: Each serving of this recipe supplies whole-food fats (2 servings).

Berry Cinnamon Pecan Muffins

Yield: 8
Total Time: 40 minutes
Prep: 15 minutes • **Cook:** 25 minutes

1⅔ cups almond flour
½ cup half pecans, chopped
6½ teaspoons cinnamon
⅓ teaspoon salt
½ cup xylitol or erythritol (optional)
1 pinch stevia
2 tablespoons solid extra–virgin coconut oil
2 large eggs (whole)
¼ cup coconut milk, unsweetened
2 teaspoons vanilla extract
2 tablespoons coconut flour

1 teaspoon baking powder
⅔ cup of your favorite berries, frozen and then thawed (blueberries or raspberries are great!)

- Preheat oven to 350°F. Prepare a muffin tin with 8 cupcake papers.
- For the topping: Combine ⅔ cup almond flour, chopped pecans, 2 tablespoons cinnamon, ⅛ teaspoon salt, 2 tablespoons xylitol or erythritol, a pinch of stevia, and 2 tablespoons melted coconut oil in a small bowl. Mix with a fork until it begins to crumble. Set aside while making the muffin batter.
- For the muffins: whisk together the eggs, coconut milk, vanilla, xylitol or erythritol, stevia, and cinnamon. Add 1 cup almond flour, coconut flour, salt, and baking powder; mix to combine, then fold in ⅔ cup berries.
- Divide into 8 muffin wells, topping each with about 2 tablespoons of the topping. Bake for 25 minutes, remove from oven, and allow to sit for 10–20 minutes to cool before removing. These may be eaten immediately or stored in an airtight container in the refrigerator for up to 1 week.

SANE Scoring: Each serving of this recipe supplies whole-food fats (1 serving).

Chocolate Chunk Bars

Yield: 8
Total Time: 30 minutes
Prep: 10 minutes • **Cook:** 20 minutes

Coconut cooking spray
¼ cup melted extra-virgin coconut oil
⅓ cup SANE honey (see below)
2 teaspoons vanilla extract
2 eggs, slightly beaten
¼ cup unsweetened almond milk
½ cup coconut flour
½ teaspoon baking soda
¼ teaspoon salt
3 ounces dark chocolate chips
½ cup unsweetened coconut flakes, optional

- Preheat oven to 350°F. Spray 8×8-inch baking pan with vegetable cooking spray.
- In a large bowl, whisk together extra-virgin coconut oil, SANE honey, vanilla, eggs, and almond milk. In a separate medium bowl, whisk together coconut flour, baking soda, and salt. Add dry ingredients to wet ingredients and mix

until just combined and batter is smooth. Fold in chocolate chips, reserving a few tablespoons for sprinkling on top if desired.

- Bake for 20–22 minutes or until edges are golden brown and knife comes out with a few crumbs attached. The batter may look like it's not all the way cooked but it will be. DO NOT OVERBAKE or it will result in dried-out bars, and no one likes that!
- Cool bars on a wire rack for at least 10 minutes so that they settle a bit, then cut into squares.

SANE Scoring: Each serving of this recipe supplies whole-food fats (1 serving).

Blueberry Cobbler

Yield: 6
Total Time: 1 hour 10 minutes
Prep: 10 minutes • **Cook:** 1 hour

3 cups washed blueberries
2 cups almond flour
¼ cup coconut flour
½ teaspoon baking soda
¼ teaspoon sea salt
½ cup SANE honey (see below)
¼ cup butter or extra-virgin olive oil spray
Drop of almond extract
3 tablespoons flax meal whisked with 9 tablespoons warm water, allowed to plump up for 5 minutes
1 tablespoon apple cider vinegar (to be added last)

- Preheat oven to 350°F.
- Spray an 8×8-inch glass dish with extra-virgin coconut oil cooking spray. Pour the blueberries into the glass dish, reserving a few berries for the top, if you wish.
- Whisk the almond and coconut flour, salt, and baking soda in a bowl. Separately, whisk together butter, SANE honey, and extract.
- Mix wet and dry ingredients together, stirring in the flax. Once well combined, quickly stir in cider vinegar. Pour batter onto berries, spreading up to the edges.
- Bake for 40–50 minutes, or until the batter is set on top.

SANE Scoring: Each serving of this recipe supplies whole-food fats (2 servings) and low-fructose fruit (1 serving).

SANE Honey

Total Time: 5 minutes
Prep: 5 minutes

½ to 1 teaspoon guar gum
¼ cup water
1½ cups erythritol

- Place ½ teaspoon guar gum, water, and erythritol in a blender or food processor. Blend completely. Add up to another ½ teaspoon of guar gum (⅛ teaspoon at a time) until you reach the desired consistency.
- Remove SANE honey using a spatula and refrigerate for at least 20 minutes before using.

Raspberry Parfait

Yield: 2
Total Time: 5 minutes
Prep: 5 minutes

½ cup coconut cream
4 ounces mascarpone
4 tablespoons xylitol
½ cup raspberries

- Beat ½ cup coconut cream until soft peaks form. Add 4 ounces mascarpone and xylitol. Beat just until smooth.
- Using ½ cup raspberries, layer with the dairy mixture in 2 parfait glasses.

SANE Scoring: Each serving of this recipe supplies whole-food fats (4 servings), low-fructose fruits (1 serving).

Almond Cookies

Yield: 24 cookies
Total Time: 20 minutes
Prep: 10 minutes • **Cook:** 10 minutes

½ cup blanched and slivered almonds
¾ cup almond flour
3 teaspoons baking powder

¾ cup xylitol
1 large egg
1 yolk of a large egg
2 teaspoons pure vanilla extract
¼ cup unsalted butter

- Preheat oven to 375°F.
- In a food processor, finely grind the almonds with the almond flour, baking powder, and xylitol. In a separate bowl with an electric mixer on medium, beat the whole egg and egg yolk, vanilla, and butter together. Fold in the almond flour by hand until just combined.
- Form the dough into 24 small balls; arrange on a baking sheet lined with parchment paper. Lightly flatten the balls to silver-dollar size.
- Bake 8–10 minutes until edges begin to brown. Let cool on the baking sheets until set, then transfer to a wire rack.

SANE Scoring: Each serving of this recipe supplies whole-food fats (1 serving).

GREEN SMOOTHIES

Blueberry Blast

Yield: 1
Total Time: 3 minutes
Prep: 3 minutes

¾ cup blueberries (frozen or fresh)
6 cups spinach
1 lemon (peeled)
½ teaspoon cinnamon
2 tablespoons superfood green powder
4 tablespoons clean whey protein (if your smoothie is a meal replacement or taken after a workout)
1 teaspoon green tea (optional)
2 tablespoons erythritol (optional)

- Add all ingredients to a high-powered blender (Vitamix is ideal) with 8 ounces of cold water and a handful of ice. Blend for 2 minutes or until completely blended (i.e., no pieces of veggies or fruit are visible). Adjust the amount of water and ice for desired consistency and desired temperature.

SANE Scoring: Each serving of this recipe supplies non-starchy vegetables (4 servings), nutrient-dense protein (1 serving, 48 grams), and low-fructose fruit (1 serving).

Coco-Cranberry Dreamsicle

Yield: 1
Total Time: 3 minutes
Prep: 3 minutes

1½ cups pitted cranberries (frozen or fresh)
3 cups mixed greens
3 cups spinach
¼ cup cocoa powder
1 lemon (peeled)
2 tablespoons erythritol (optional)
½ teaspoon cinnamon
1–3 tablespoons superfood green powder
4 tablespoons clean whey protein or pea protein (if your smoothie is a
    meal replacement or taken after a workout)

- Add all ingredients to a high-powered blender with 8 ounces cold water and a handful of ice. Blend for 2 minutes or until completely blended (i.e., no pieces of veggies or fruit are visible). Adjust water and ice for desired consistency and temperature.

SANE Scoring: Each serving of this recipe supplies non-starchy vegetables (4 servings), nutrient-dense protein (1 serving, 48 grams), and low-fructose fruit (1 serving).

Grapefruit Magic

Yield: 1
Total Time: 3 minutes
Prep: 3 minutes

1 medium grapefruit (peeled)
2 cups arugula
4 cups spinach
1 lemon (peeled)

½ teaspoon cinnamon
2 tablespoons superfood green powder
4 tablespoons clean whey protein
1 teaspoon healing green tea
2 tablespoons erythritol (optional)

- Add all ingredients to a high-powered blender (Vitamix is ideal) with 8 ounces cold water and a handful of ice. Blend for 2 minutes or until completely blended (i.e., no pieces of veggies or fruit are visible). Adjust the amount of water and ice for desired consistency and desired temperature.

SANE Scoring: Each serving of this recipe supplies non-starchy vegetables (4 servings), nutrient-dense protein (1 serving, 48 grams), and low-fructose fruit (1 serving).

APPENDIX B

Diabesity: The Hidden Epidemic That's 19 Percent More Deadly Than Cancer

Going SANE is about so much more than dropping dress and pants sizes. It's about so much more than being free of the manipulative clutches of the dieting and weight-loss industry. Going SANE is about lifelong protection from the most common and deadly disease facing the world today: diabesity, the condition in which you suffer from both type 2 diabetes and obesity simultaneously.

Whether you have heard this called "diabesity" or not, it's essential for both you and your loved ones that you know how massive and tragic a problem diabesity is. Impacting more than a billion people worldwide, including 50 percent of Americans over 65, it is the largest health epidemic in human history, according to a 2017 report published in *Clinical Diabetes and Endocrinology* (Zimmet 2017).

Diabesity is especially relevant to us because both obesity and type 2 diabetes are symptoms of an elevated setpoint. And sadly, obesity leads to type 2 diabetes, and vice versa. In fact, if someone has obesity, there is a 90 percent chance they will develop type 2 diabetes. To put that in perspective, someone who smokes for 30 years has about a 10 percent chance of developing lung cancer.

While we don't yet know why the brain, gut, and hormonal issues at the heart of an elevated setpoint show up first as type 2 diabetes in some people and as obesity in others, we do know that when one shows up, the other is soon to follow. Here's how this works from a high level in both cases: A diagnosis of type 2 diabetes means insulin is building up in your bloodstream. This makes it almost impossible for your body to burn stored fat for fuel. That makes obesity almost inevitable. Similarly, a diagnosis of obesity means your brain, gut, hormones, or all of them can't do their job. This leads to insulin building up in your bloodstream, which leads to type 2 diabetes.

So if your brain, gut, and/or hormones are not healthy, your setpoint will rise and if nothing is done, you will be diagnosed with either obesity or type 2

diabetes. Then, if nothing is done after that diagnosis, the other diagnosis *will* follow, and you will have diabesity. Having diabesity means your metabolic system,
which includes your brain, gut, and hormones, is so broken that you are at very
high risk of heart disease, stroke, dementia, Alzheimer's, cancer, high blood pressure, amputation, blindness, and kidney failure. I know this sounds terrible, but
that's because it is. What is even more outrageous is that traditional health care
attempts to treat this condition with the "eat less, exercise more" mythology that
we know only makes matters worse! When your brain, gut, and hormones all
can't do their jobs, the body will not be able to do anything for much longer, and
your life expectancy will drop by about 29 years.

I do not want this for you. I know YOU certainly don't want this for you.
I know your children, grandchildren, relatives, and friends want you around as
long as possible. And I know you want the same for them. So here's the key: *Every-
body* can avoid this! Diabesity is both 100 percent preventable and reversible with
doable and sustainable lifestyle changes. SANE eating, exercise, and living are
among the most potent medicines to heal and protect your brain, gut, and hormones. For example…

One of SANE's most powerful case studies regarding diabesity is Sam, 68,
a construction manager and former NFL player with the San Francisco 49ers.
Sam had been overweight all his life, except during his stint in pro football. But
throughout the rest of his life, he struggled with obesity and was the classic yo-yo
dieter, going up and down 100 to 200 pounds at any given time. Like most dieters, Sam tried everything, including lap band surgery that failed and almost cost
him his life. By early 2016, he was obese again, nearly 120 pounds over a healthy
weight.

In May 2017, Sam received what he referred to as a "death sentence": type 2
diabetes. Sam knew the consequences; his older brother had his leg amputated as
a result of diabetes. Sam's was a classic case of diabesity: diabetes brought on by
obesity. He was immediately put on the oral diabetes drug metformin.

Sam was determined to defeat his diabetes—and lose weight once and for all.
He embarked on a calorie-counting diet that included oatmeal, grapes, watermelon, fiber bars, and occasionally packaged food from Nutrisystem—all of
which he thought would help him lose weight and get healthy. Well, he was losing
weight, but only at the rate of a pound or half a pound a week—extremely slow for
a man. It was frustrating.

Enter his fiancée, Maggie Greenwood-Robinson, author of *Control Diabetes in 6 Easy Steps* and *Foods That Combat Diabetes*; a series of Biggest Loser books; and a collaborator on countless diet books (including this one). To say that she is familiar with most diet plans would be an understatement.

Maggie started working with the SANE team in September 2017. She was instantly amazed by the program. "I thought I knew just about everything there is to know about food and weight control, but SANE opened my eyes to new information...strategies and concepts such as standard carbohydrates and how nonessential they are; the importance of whole-food fats, setpoint science, hormonal influences on weight; the fallacy of calorie counting; and so much more."

Maggie put Sam on SANE right away. Pretty soon, Sam was dropping 4 to 5 pounds a week—consistently. No more oatmeal for breakfast—it was egg-white-and-veggie omelets. Gone were the high-sugar grapes and watermelon; in their place were blueberries on occasion. Sam never strayed from SANE. He felt so good about the plan that he told everyone, "I love losing weight on SANE."

By February 2018, he had dropped 85 pounds. But that's not all. The best news came from his doctor, who proclaimed him cured of diabetes and took him off metformin immediately. "In 35 years of practicing medicine, I have never seen anything like this," said Sam's doctor.

When Sam hit a loss of 105 pounds through SANE living, he went "shopping in his closet." This involved tossing out all fat clothes and rediscovering clothes he had not worn in years. He found 36 pairs of pants, two sport coats, 34 shirts, and three suits that now fit—where they did not before.

Then, by the first week of July 2018, Sam had dropped a total of 170 pounds. The good news kept coming. Sam had his annual eye exam. An optometrist can do certain tests of your eyes and see if you have conditions such as type 2 diabetes. After the eye doctor peered into Sam's eyes via electronic tests, it was confirmed: no diabetes!

"Most people who are diagnosed with type 2 diabetes take their medicine but never really change their diet," Maggie emphasized. "As a result, they often escalate to taking a second drug and sometimes have to go on insulin. None of this has to happen. The SANE nutritional plan has the power to stop diabetes and diabesity completely. It should be the standard, first-line approach for treating these twin epidemics, in my opinion, not drugs. It is miraculous in its effect, and Sam is living proof." To help protect yourself and your loved ones from diabesity, get started by taking this quiz to determine your risk.

Diabesity Quiz

1. Are you more than 40 pounds over your ideal or healthy weight?

    ☐ Yes ☐ No

    For a "yes" answer, give yourself 10 points: _____

    For a "no" answer, give yourself 0 points: _____

    Fact: For every 2.2 pounds of weight you gain, your risk of diabetes increases
    by 4.5 percent, says a 2013 report published in the *Journal of the Pakistan
    Medical Association* and other medical journals—which is why losing
    weight is the most commonly prescribed way to prevent and reverse
    diabesity (Kaira 2013). But as you and I know, the traditional "eat less
    and exercise more" model just makes things worse!

2. Has your doctor told you that your blood sugar has been consistently
    higher than 126, or that your hemoglobin A1C is greater than 6.5, which
    is diabetes?

    ☐ Yes ☐ No

    For a "yes" answer, give yourself 10 points: _____

    For a "no" answer, give yourself 0 points: _____

    Fact: Hyperglycemia, having high blood sugar levels, is telling of insulin
    resistance. While insulin resistance can be characteristic of both obesity
    and diabetes, you do not have to be currently obese to suffer insulin
    resistance and type 2 diabetes.

3. Is your waist measurement 40 inches or more (for men) or more than 35
    inches (for women)?

    ☐ Yes ☐ No

    For a "yes" answer, give yourself 7 points: _____

    For a "no" answer, give yourself 0 points: _____

    Fact: Studies suggest that abdominal fat causes fat cells to release pro-
    inflammatory chemicals that promote insulin resistance, making both
    obesity and type 2 diabetes worse. Belly fat is considered a risk factor
    for diabesity.

4. Do you have a family history of type 2 diabetes or obesity?

    ☐ Yes ☐ No

    For a "yes" answer, give yourself 4 points: _____

    For a "no" answer, give yourself 0 points: _____

Fact: There is a genetic basis for both—although heredity is not destiny when it comes to preventing and reversing both conditions. A SANE diet and other healthy lifestyle choices can react positively with your unique genetic tendencies.

5. Have there been periods of time in your life when most of your meals consisted of 2 or more servings of starches such as bread, cereal, pasta, rice, corn, or potatoes?

☐ Yes ☐ No

For a "yes" answer, give yourself 4 points: _____

For a "no" answer, give yourself 0 points: _____

Fact: When your diet is full of non-vegetable carbohydrates over time, your cells become resistant or insensitive to the effects of insulin, leading to insulin resistance. A higher insulin level is a key indicator of diabesity; your physician can test you for high insulin and hemoglobin A1C.

6. Have there been periods in your life when you habitually drank more than one sugar-laden beverage per day such as juice, sodas, punches, energy drinks, or sweetened coffee?

For a "yes" answer, give yourself 4 points: _____

For a "no" answer, give yourself 0 points: _____

Fact: Sugar-sweetened beverages are the single largest source of added sugar and the top source of energy intake in the U.S. diet, according to a report published in 2013 in *Obesity Reviews* (Hu 2013). This report is among several scientific articles citing evidence that avoiding such beverages will decrease the risk of obesity and related diseases such as diabetes.

7. Do you have trouble losing weight on a diet, or does weight come off very slowly when you diet?

☐ Yes ☐ No

For a "yes" answer, give yourself 3 points: _____

For a "no" answer, give yourself 0 points: _____

Fact: People with diabesity, and those at risk for developing diabesity, find it relatively difficult to lose weight and burn fat. An obese person with diabetes can lose only half as much body weight as someone who is overweight or obese but does not have diabetes. Why the discrepancy?

Insulin resistance makes it tough for a diabese person to lose weight, because of insulin's effect on setpoint.

8. Has your doctor told you that you have a low level of HDL cholesterol (50 mg/dL or less if male, or 60 mg/dL or less if female)?

☐ Yes ☐ No

For a "yes" answer, give yourself 3 points: _____

For a "no" answer, give yourself 0 points: _____

Fact: Insulin resistance is associated with lowering HDL cholesterol (the good cholesterol). (The higher your HDL cholesterol, the better it is for your heart health.) Not everyone with low HDL, however, has diabesity.

9. Has your doctor told you that you have a triglyceride level of 100 mg/Dl or higher?

☐ Yes ☐ No

For a "yes" answer, give yourself 3 points: _____

For a "no" answer, give yourself 0 points: _____

Fact: Triglycerides are blood fats associated with abdominal obesity, diabetes, diabesity, insulin resistance, and low levels of HDL cholesterol. Elevated triglycerides are a possible sign of diabesity. Not everyone with elevated triglycerides, however, has diabesity.

10. Has your doctor told you that you have high blood pressure?

☐ Yes ☐ No

For a "yes" answer, give yourself 3 points: _____

For a "no" answer, give yourself 0 points: _____

Fact: A condition associated with insulin resistance is high blood pressure—which is why hypertension is considered a symptom of diabesity. Not everyone with hypertension, however, has diabesity.

11. Do you get little or no exercise through the week?

☐ Yes ☐ No

For a "yes" answer, give yourself 3 points: _____

For a "no" answer, give yourself 0 points: _____

Fact: Certain forms of exercise, including walking and resistance training, help the body's muscle cells become more receptive to insulin, thereby preventing insulin resistance. "Smart" exercise, the form you learned in this book, will actually contribute to reversing insulin resistance.

Scoring:

Look at your points for each question and add them up. The higher your score, the higher your risk. Generally, if you scored between 31 and 50, you either have diabesity or are about to. Please visit your doctor and Go SANE immediately and intensely. If your score is between 20 and 30, you have a high risk of developing diabesity if you don't have it already. Please put SANEity and lowering your setpoint at the top of your to-do list for this month. If you scored between 10 and 19, be sure to Go SANE to keep a diabesity diagnosis at bay. You are in pretty good shape, and you deserve to stay that way. If you scored below 9, chances are you said "I do that already" a lot while reading this book because your low setpoint and SANE lifestyle are already keeping diabesity at bay. Keep it up!

I'd imagine that if you took this quiz after reading this entire book, you don't need any more motivation to Go SANE and lower your setpoint by healing your brain, gut, and hormones. However, sometimes quantifying risk can provide that extra push that keeps you going in those dark moments when lifestyle change is especially hard. The key is that regardless of your risk, you now have access to the most potent therapeutic protocol to prevent or reverse the diabesity, and, one more time, that's awesome.

Disclaimer: This assessment is for informational purposes only. It is not meant to diagnose any condition or illness. For questions, diagnoses, and treatment for diabetes, obesity, or diabesity, please consult your physician.

APPENDIX C

Next Steps and SANE Solution Resources

Our deepest fear is not that we are inadequate. Our deepest fear is that we are powerful beyond measure. It is our light, not our darkness, that most frightens us. We ask ourselves: Who am I to be brilliant, gorgeous, talented, and fabulous? Actually, who are you not to be?...Your playing small does not serve the world. There is nothing enlightened about shrinking so that other people will not feel insecure around you. We are all meant to shine...and as we let our own light shine, we unconsciously give others permission to do the same. As we are liberated from our own fear, our presence automatically liberates others.

—Marianne Williamson

In the past, the "truth" about our body, mind, and spirit has been determined by a number of factors, including toxic media messages and disempowering market forces. This no longer has to be the case. The truth is beautiful, and so are you. We simply need to get the word out. If every one of us spends a few seconds sharing this proven science, these practical habits, and this powerful love, we can create a healthier and happier world. Any help you would be willing to provide to share the SANEity would be deeply appreciated.

In support of these messages, I host several free online events and I'd love to meet you there. You can learn about these events and health topics, and you can get meal plans, recipe books, food lists, how-to videos, cheat sheets, step-by-step guides, trackers, journals, and more at SANESolution.com.

SELECTED BIBLIOGRAPHY

Full bibliography available at: https://SANESolution.com/bibliography

INTRODUCTION

Andreyeva, T., et al. "Changes in perceived weight discrimination among Americans, 1995–1996 through 2004–2006." *Obesity* 16 (2008):1129–34.

Aubrey, A. "Is dieting passé? Study finds fewer overweight people try to lose weight." *Salt* (March 8, 2017).

Puhl, R.M., and Heurer, C.A. "Obesity stigma: Important considerations for public health." *American Journal of Public Health* 100 (2010): 1019–28.

Rand, C.S., and MacGregor, A.M. "Successful weight loss following obesity surgery and the perceived liability of morbid obesity." *International Journal of Obesity* 15 (1991): 577–79.

Sifferlin, A. "The weight loss trap: Why your diet isn't working." *Time* (May 25, 2017).

Wild, S., et al. "Global prevalence of diabetes: Estimates for the year 2000 and projections for 2030." *Diabetes Care* 27 (2004): 1047–53.

"World population estimates," Wikipedia, https://en.wikipedia.org/wiki/World_population_estimates#Before_1950.

Zimmet, P. "Diabesity—the biggest epidemic in human history." *Medscape General Medicine* 9 (2007): 39.

CHAPTER 1: UNLOCK THE NATURALLY THIN YOU

Crawford, D., et al. "Can anyone successfully control their weight? Findings of a three year community-based study of men and women." *International Journal of Obesity Related Metabolic Disorders* 24 (2000): 1107–10.

Fothergill, E., et al. "Persistent metabolic adaptation 6 years after 'The Biggest Loser' competition." *Obesity* 24 (2016): 1612–19.

Garner, D.M., and Wooley, S.C. "Confronting the failure of behavioral and dietary treatments for obesity." *Clinical Psychology Review* 11 (1991): 729–80.

Keys, A., et al. *The Biology of Human Starvation*. 2 vols. St. Paul, MN: University of Minnesota Press, 1950.

Krieger, J.W., et al. "Effects of variation in protein and carbohydrate intake on body mass and composition during energy restriction: a meta-regression." *American Journal of Clinical Nutrition* 83 (2006): 260–74.

Leibel, R.L., and Hirsch, J. "Diminished energy requirements in reduced-obese patients." *Metabolism* 33 (1984): 164–70.

Leibel, R.L., et al. "Changes in energy expenditure resulting from altered body weight." *New England Journal of Medicine* 332 (1995): 621–28.

Levine, J.A., et al. "Role of nonexercise activity thermogenesis in resistance to fat gain in humans." *Science* 283 (1999): 212–14.

Ley, S.H., et al. "Prevention and management of type 2 diabetes: Dietary components and nutritional strategies." *Lancet* 383 (2014): 1999–2007.

Lyon, D.M., and Dunlop, D.M. "The treatment of obesity: A comparison of the effects of diet and of thyroid extract." *Quarterly Journal of Medicine* 1 (1932): 331–52.

Lyon, H.N., and Hirschhorn, J.N. "Genetics of common forms of obesity: A brief overview." *American Journal of Clinical Nutrition* 82 (2005): 215S–17S.

Maclean, P.S., et al. "Enhanced metabolic efficiency contributes to weight regain after weight loss in obesity-prone rats." *American Journal of Physiology* 287 (2004): R1306–15.

Puhl, R.M., and Heurer, C.A. "Obesity stigma: Important considerations for public health." *American Journal of Public Health*. 100 (2010): 1019–28.

Weigle, D.S. "Human obesity: Exploding the myths." *West Journal of Medicine* 153 (1990): 421–28.

Young, E.A., et al. "Hepatic response to a very-low-energy diet and refeeding in rats." *American Journal of Clinical Nutrition* 57 (1993): 857–62.

CHAPTER 2: THE THREE HIDDEN FACTORS THAT DETERMINE YOUR WEIGHT

Farias, M.M., et al. "Set-point theory and obesity." *Metabolic Syndrome and Related Disorders* 9 (2011): 85–89.

Kadooka, Y., et al. "Regulation of abdominal adiposity by probiotics (*Lactobacillus gasseri* SBT2055) in adults with obese tendencies in a randomized controlled trial." *European Journal of Clinical Nutrition* 64 (2010): 636–43.

Million, M., et al. "Gut bacterial microbiota and obesity." *Clinical Microbiology and Infection* 19 (2013): 305–13.

Rezzi, S., et al. "Human metabolic phenotypes link directly to specific dietary preferences in healthy individuals." *Journal of Proteome Research* 6 (2007): 4469–77.

Ridaura, V.K., et al. "Gut microbiota from twins discordant for obesity modulate metabolism in mice." *Science* 341 (2013): 124214.

Sanchez, M., et al. "Effect of *Lactobacillus rhamnosus* CGMCC1.3724 supplementation on weight loss and maintenance in obese men and women." *British Journal of Nutrition* 111 (2014): 1507–19.

Thaler, J.P., et al. "Obesity is associated with hypothalamic injury in rodents and humans." *Journal of Clinical Investigation* 122 (2012): 153–62.

Viggiano, E., et al. "Effects of a high-fat diet enriched in lard or in fish oil on the hypothalamic amp-activated protein kinase and inflammatory mediators." *Frontiers in Cellular Neuroscience* 10 (2016): 150.

CHAPTER 3: GOOD CALORIES, BAD CALORIES, AND SANE CALORIES...OH MY!

Barkeling, B., et al. Effects of a high-protein meal (meat) and a high-carbohydrate meal (vegetarian) on satiety measured by automated computerized monitoring of subsequent food intake, motivation to eat and food preferences. *International Journal of Obesity* 14 (1990): 743–51.

Boden, G., et al. "Effect of a low-carbohydrate diet on appetite, blood glucose levels, and insulin resistance in obese patients with type 2 diabetes." *Annals of Internal Medicine* 142 (2005): 403–11.

Booth, D.A., et al. "Relative effectiveness of protein in the late stages of appetite suppression in man." *Physiology & Behavior* 5 (1970): 1299–1302.

Halton, T.L., and Hu, F.B. "The effects of high protein diets on thermogenesis, satiety and weight loss: A critical review." *Journal of the American College of Nutrition* 23 (2004): 373–85.

Hill, A.J., and Blundell, J.E. "Macronutrients and satiety: The effects of a high protein or high carbohydrate meal on subjective motivation to eat and food preferences." *Nutrition and Behavior* 3 (1986): 133–44.

Kadey, M. "A nutrient-dense diet delivers optimal health." *Environmental Nutrition* (February 28, 2015).

Raymond, J. "Filling up with less." *Newsweek* (March 19, 2007).

Weigle, D.S., et al. "A high-protein diet induces sustained reductions in appetite, ad libitum caloric intake, and body weight despite compensatory changes in diurnal plasma leptin and ghrelin concentrations." *American Journal of Clinical Nutrition* 82 (2005): 41–48.

CHAPTER 4: NON-STARCHY VEGETABLES

Carter, P., et al. "Fruit and vegetable intake and incidence of type 2 diabetes mellitus: Systematic review and meta-analysis." *BMJ* 341 (2010): c4229.

Kahn, H.S., et al. "Stable behaviors associated with adults' 10-year change in body mass index and likelihood of gain at the waist." *American Journal of Public Health* 87 (1997): 747–54.

Reiss, R., et al. "Estimation of cancer risks and benefits associated with a potential increased consumption of fruits and vegetables." *Journal of Food and Chemical Toxicology* 50 (2012): 4421–27.

CHAPTER 5: NUTRIENT-DENSE PROTEINS

Cordain, Loren, PhD, and Campbell, T. Colin, PhD. "The Protein Debate," www .catalystathletics.com/articles/downloads/proteinDebate.pdf.

Layman, D.K. University of Illinois at Urbana-Champaign, Department of Food Science, personal communications.

Masterjohn, C. The curious case of Campbell's rats—does protein deficiency prevent cancer? Weston A. Price Foundation, published online September, 22, 2010, https://www.westonaprice.org/the-curious-case-of-campbells-rats-does-protein -deficiency-prevent-cancer/

Willett, W.C., and Hu, F.B. "Optimal diets for prevention of coronary heart disease." *Journal of the American Medical Association* 288 (2002): 2578–69.

CHAPTER 6: WHOLE-FOOD FATS AND SWEETS

Berryman, C.E., et al. "Effects of daily almond consumption on cardiometabolic risk and abdominal adiposity in healthy adults with elevated LDL-cholesterol: A randomized controlled trial." *Journal of the American Heart Association* 4 (2015): e000993.

Dreher, M.L., and Davenport, A.J. "Hass avocado composition and potential health effects." *Critical Reviews in Food Science and Nutrition* 53 (2013): 738–50.

Hu, F.B., et al. "Types of dietary fat and risk of coronary heart disease: a critical review." *Journal of the American College of Nutrition* 20 (2001): 5–19.

Ludwig, D.S. "Lowering the bar on the low-fat diet." *Journal of the American Medical Association* 316 (2016): 2087–88.

Parks, E.J., et al. "Dietary sugars stimulate fatty acid synthesis in adults." *Journal of Nutrition* 138 (2008): 1039–46.

Shapiro, A., et al. "Fructose-induced leptin resistance exacerbates weight gain in response to subsequent high-fat feeding." *American Journal of Physiology-Regulatory, Integrative, and Comparative Physiology* 295 (2008): R1370–R1375.

Singer, G.M., and Geohas, J. "The effect of chromium picolinate and biotin supplementation on glycemic control in poorly controlled patients with type 2 diabetes mellitus: A placebo-controlled, double-blinded, randomized trial." *Diabetes Technology & Therapeutics* 8 (2006): 5–19.

Smith, C. E., et al. "Dietary fatty acids modulate associations between genetic variants and circulating fatty acids in plasma and erythrocyte membranes: meta-analysis of nine studies in the CHARGE consortium." *Molecular Nutrition and Food Research* 59 (2015): 1373–83.

Wutzke, K.D., and Lorenz, H. "The effect of l-carnitine on fat oxidation, protein turnover, and body composition in slightly overweight subjects." *Metabolism* 53 (2004): 1002–6.

Zahedi, H., et al. "Effects of CoQ10 supplementation on lipid profiles and glycemic control in patients with type 2 diabetes: a randomized, double blind, placebo-controlled trial." *Journal of Diabetes and Metabolic Disorders* 13 (2004): 81.

CHAPTER 7: SMOOTHIES AND BEVERAGES

Chen, I.J., et al. "Therapeutic effect of high-dose green tea extract on weight reduction: A randomized, double-blind, placebo-controlled clinical trial." *Clinical Nutrition* 35 (2016): 592–99.

Johnson, C.S., and Gaas, C.A. "Vinegar: medicinal uses and antiglycemic effect." *Medscape General Medicine* 8 (2006): 61.

Keithley, J., and Swanson, B. "Glucomannan and obesity: A critical review." *Alternative Therapies in Health and Medicine* 11 (2005): 30–34.

Kumar, S., et al. "A double-blind, placebo-controlled, randomised, clinical study on the effectiveness of collagen peptide on osteoarthritis." *Journal of the Science of Food and Agriculture* 95 (2015): 702–07.

Liu, D., et al. "Collagen and gelatin." *Annual Review of Food Science and Technology* 6 (2015): 527–57.

Li, Y., et al. "Effects of tea or tea extract on metabolic profiles in patients with type 2 diabetes mellitus: A meta-analysis of ten randomized controlled trials." *Diabetes/Metabolism Research and Reviews* 32 (2016): 2–10.

Ohashi, Y., et al. "Consumption of partially hydrolysed guar gum stimulates Bifidobacteria and butyrate-producing bacteria in the human large intestine." *Beneficial Microbes* 6 (2015): 451–55.

Ranasinghe, P., et al. "Medicinal properties of 'true' cinnamon (*Cinnamomum zeylanicum*): A systematic review." *BMC Complementary and Alternative Medicine* 13 (2013): 275.

Rao, T.P. "Role of guar fiber in appetite control." *Physiology & Behavior* 164 (Part A; 2016): 277–83.

CHAPTER 8: MEAL PLANNING FOR A LOWER SETPOINT

Pelchat, M.L., and Schaefer, S. "Dietary monotony and food cravings in young and elderly adults." *Physiology & Behavior* 68 (2000): 353–59.

Vishton, Peter M., PhD. "Outsmart Yourself: Brain-Based Strategies to a Better You," https://www.thegreatcourses.com/courses/outsmart-yourself-brain-based -strategies-to-a-better-you.html.

CHAPTER 9: COOKING AND EVERY RECIPE YOU'LL EVER NEED

[no resources]

CHAPTER 10: DIET PILLS, BAD. NUTRACEUTICALS, GOOD.

Best, C.H., et al. "The rates of lipotropic action of choline and inositol under special dietary conditions." *Biochemical Journal* 48 (1951): 452–58.

Bortolotti, M., et al. "Effects of a whey protein supplementation on intrahepatocellular lipids in obese female patients." *Clinical Nutrition* 30 (2011): 494–98.

Bowen, J., et al. "Appetite hormones and energy intake in obese men after consumption of fructose, glucose and whey protein beverages." *International Journal of Obesity* 31 (2007): 1696–1703.

Broadhurst, C.L., and Domenico, P. "Clinical studies on chromium picolinate supplementation in diabetes mellitus—a review." *Diabetes Technology & Therapeutics* 8 (2006): 677–87.

Cheang, K.I., et al. "Effect on insulin-stimulated release of d-chiro-inositol-containing inositolphosphoglycan mediator during weight loss in obese women with and without polycystic ovary syndrome." *International Journal of Endocrinology* (2016).

Cholewa, J.M., et al. "Effects of betaine and body composition: A review of recent findings and potential mechanisms." *Amino Acids* 46 (2014): 1785–93.

Chungchunlam, S.M., et al. "Dietary whey protein influences plasma satiety-related hormones and plasma amino acids in normal-weight adult women." *European Journal of Clinical Nutrition* 69 (2015): 179–86.

De Souza, A.Z., et al. "Oral supplementation with L-glutamine alters gut microbiota of obese and overweight adults: A pilot study." *Nutrition* 31 (2015): 884–89.

Docherty, J.P., et al. "A double-blind, placebo-controlled, exploratory trial of chromium picolinate in atypical depression: Effect on carbohydrate craving." *Journal of Psychiatric Practice* 11 (2005): 302–14.

Gao, X., et al. "Higher dietary choline and betaine intakes are associated with better body composition in the adult population of Newfoundland, Canada." *PLOS One* 11 (2016): e0155403.

Garrido-Maraver, J., et al. "Clinical applications of coenzyme Q10." *Frontiers in Bioscience* 19 (2014): 619–33.

Iscoc, K.E., et al. "Efficacy of continuous real-time blood glucose monitoring during and after prolonged high-intensity cycling exercise: Spinning with a continuous glucose monitoring system." *Diabetes Technology & Therapeutics* 8 (2006): 627–35.

Kabadi, S.M., et al. "Joint effects of obesity and vitamin D insufficiency on insulin resistance and type 2 diabetes: Results from the NHANES 2001–2006." *Diabetes Care* 35 (2012): 2048–54.

Kadooka, Y., et al. "Regulation of abdominal adiposity by probiotics (*Lactobacillus gasseri* SBT2055) in adults with obese tendencies in a randomized controlled trial." *European Journal of Clinical Nutrition* 64 (2010): 636–43.

Layman, D.K., et al. "A reduced ratio of dietary carbohydrate to protein improves body composition and blood lipid profiles during weight loss in adult women." *Journal of Nutrition* 133 (2003): 411–17.

Manna, P., et al. "Role of sulfur containing amino acids as an adjuvant therapy in the prevention of diabetes and its associated complications." *Current Diabetes Reviews* 9 (2013): 237–48.

Parker, J., et al. "Levels of vitamin D and cardiometabolic disorders: Systematic review and meta-analysis." *Maturitas* 65 (2009): 225–36.

Parnell, J.A., and Reimer, R.A. "Weight loss during oligofructose supplementation is associated with decreased ghrelin and increased peptide YY in overweight and obese adults." *American Journal of Clinical Nutrition* 89 (2009): 1751–59.

Patel, S. "Emerging trends in nutraceutical applications of whey protein and its derivatives." *Journal of Food Science and Technology* 52 (2015): 6847–58.

Samimi, M., et al. "Oral carnitine supplementation reduced body weight and insulin resistance in women with polycystic ovary syndrome: A randomized, double-blind, placebo-controlled trial." *Clinical Endocrinology* 84 (2016): 851–57.

Smith, A.D., and Refsum, H. "Vitamin B-12 and cognition in the elderly." *American Journal of Clinical Nutrition* 89 (2009): 707S–711S.

Verrusio, W., et al. "Association between serum vitamin D and metabolic syndrome in middle-aged and older adults and role of supplementation therapy with vitamin D." *Annali dell'Istituto Superiore di Sanità* 53 (2017): 54–59.

Wang, Z.Q. "Chromium picolinate enhances skeletal muscle cellular insulin signaling in vivo in obese, insulin-resistant JCR:LA-cp rats." *Journal of Nutrition* 136 (2006): 415–20.

CHAPTER 11: EXERCISE LESS, LOWER YOUR SETPOINT MORE

Arciero, P.J., et al. "Increased dietary protein and combined high intensity aerobic and resistance exercise improves body fat distribution and cardiovascular risk factors." *International Journal of Sports Nutrition and Exercise Metabolism* 16 (2006): 373–92.

Earnest, C.P. "Exercise interval training: an improved stimulus for improving the physiology of pre-diabetes." *Medical Hypotheses* 71 (2008): 752–61.

Friedman, J.M. "Modern science versus the stigma of obesity." *Nature Medicine* 10 (2004): 563–69.

Hortobagvi, T., et al. "The effects of detraining on power athletes." *Medicine & Science in Sports & Exercise* 25 (1993): 929–35.

Irving, B.A., et al. "Effect of exercise training intensity on abdominal visceral fat and body composition." *Medicine & Science in Sports & Exercise* 40 (2008): 1863–72.

Izumiya, Y., et al. "Fast/glycolytic muscle fiber growth reduces fat mass and improves metabolic parameters in obese mice." *Cell Metabolism* 7 (2008): 159–72.

Kolata, G.B. *Ultimate Fitness: The Quest for Truth about Exercise and Health.* New York: Farrar, Straus and Giroux, 2003.

Ludwig, D.S., and Friedman, M.I. "Increasing adiposity: Consequence or cause of overeating?" *Journal of the American Medical Association* 311 (2014): 2167–68.

McGuff, D. and Little, J.R. *Body by Science: A Research Based Program to Get the Results You Want in 12 Minutes a Week.* New York: McGraw-Hill, 2009.

Murray, C.J.L., et al. "Obesity continues to rise in nearly all countries but Americans becoming more physically active, too." Published by the Institute for Health Metrics and Evaluation at www.healthdata.org/node/1640, July 10, 2013.

Ormsbee, M.J., et al. "Fat metabolism and acute resistance exercise in trained men." *Journal of Applied Physiology* 102 (2007): 1767–72.

Paschalis, V., et al. "A weekly bout of eccentric exercise is sufficient to induce health-promoting effects." *Medicine & Science in Sports & Exercise* 43 (2011): 64–73.

CHAPTER 12: THE 20-MINUTE-PER-WEEK SANE EXERCISE PROGRAM

Sim, A.Y., et al. "Effects of high-intensity intermittent exercise training on appetite regulation." *Medicine & Science in Sports & Exercise* 47 (2015): 2441–49.

CHAPTER 13: LOVE YOURSELF SLIM

Adams, C., and Leary, M. "Promoting self-compassionate attitudes toward eating among restrictive and guilty eaters." *Journal of Social and Clinical Psychology* 26 (2007): 1120–44.

Armitage, C., et al. "Randomized controlled trial of a volitional help sheet to encourage weight loss in the Middle East." *Prevention Science* 18 (2017): 976–83.

Luszczynska, A., et al. "Planning to lose weight: Randomized controlled trial of an implementation intention prompt to enhance weight reduction among overweight and obese women." *Health Psychology* 26 (2007): 507–12.

CHAPTER 14: SIMPLE SETPOINT-LOWERING HABITS

Gearhardt, A.N., et al. "Preliminary validation of the Yale Food Addiction Scale." *Appetite* 52 (2009): 430–36.

Hwang, K.O., et al. "Social Support in an Internet Weight Loss Community." *International Journal of Medical Information* 79 (2010): 5–13.

Kelley, A.E., et al. "Opioid modulation of taste hedonics within the ventral striatum." *Physiology & Behavior* 76 (2002): 365–77.

McCullough, M.E., Emmons, R.A., and Tsang, J.A. "The grateful disposition: A conceptual and empirical topography." *Journal of Personality and Social Psychology* 82 (2002): 112–27.

Segerstrom, S.C., and Nes, L.S. "Heart rate variability reflects self-regulatory strength, effort, and fatigue." *Psychological Science* 18 (2007): 275–81.

Verheijden, M.W., et al. "Role of social support in lifestyle-focused weight management interventions." *European Journal of Clinical Nutrition* 59 Supplement 1 (2005): 179–86.

CHAPTER 15: THE 21-DAY SANE SETPOINT SOLUTION

Albertson, E.R., et al. "Self-compassion and body dissatisfaction in women: A randomized controlled trial of a brief meditation intervention." *Mindfulness* (2014). doi:10.1007/s12671-014-0277-3.

Hollis, J.F., et al. "Weight loss during the intensive intervention phase of the weight-loss maintenance trial." *American Journal of Preventive Medicine* 35 (2008): 118–26.

CHAPTER 16: #SANE4LIFE

Barrea. L., et al. "Low serum vitamin D-status, air pollution and obesity: A dangerous liaison." *Reviews in Endocrine and Metabolic Disorders* 18 (2017): 207–14.

Kristal, A.R., et al. "Yoga practice is associated with attenuated weight gain in healthy, middle-aged men and women." *Alternative Therapies in Health and Medicine* 11 (2005): 28–33.

Muscogiuri, G., et al. "Obesogenic endocrine disruptors and obesity: Myths and truths." *Archives of Toxicology* 91 (2017): 3469–75.

APPENDIX A: SANE SETPOINT-LOWERING RECIPES

[no resources]

APPENDIX B: DIABESITY: THE HIDDEN EPIDEMIC THAT'S 19 PERCENT MORE DEADLY THAN CANCER

Hu, F.B. "Resolved: there is sufficient scientific evidence that decreasing sugar-sweetened beverage consumption will reduce the prevalence of obesity and obesity-related disease." *Obesity Reviews* 14 (2013): 606–19.

Kaira, S. "Diabesity." *Journal of the Pakistan Medical Association* 63 (2013): 532–34.

Zimmet, P.Z. "Diabetes and its drivers: the largest epidemic in human history?" *Clinical Diabetes and Endocrinology* 18 (2017): 1.

APPENDIX C: NEXT STEPS AND SANE SOLUTION RESOURCES

[no resources]

INDEX

ABOUT THE AUTHOR

Jonathan Bailor pioneered the field of Wellness Engineering and is the founder and CEO of the world's fastest-growing permanent weight loss and diabesity treatment company, SANESolution. He authored the *New York Times* best seller *The Calorie Myth*, has registered over 26 patents, has spoken at Fortune 100 companies and TED conferences for over a decade, and has served as a Senior Program Manager at Microsoft, where he helped create Nike+ Kinect Training and Xbox Fitness. His work has been endorsed and implemented by top doctors from Harvard Medical School, Johns Hopkins, the Mayo Clinic, the Cleveland Clinic, and UCLA. A summa cum laude and Phi Beta Kappa graduate of DePauw University, Bailor lives outside Seattle with his wife, Angela, and daughter, Aavia Gabrielle. Learn more at SANESolution.com.